Study Guide to accompany Christensen & Kockrow

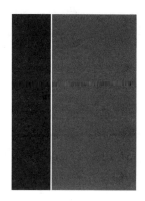

Foundations of Nursing

Fourth Edition

Patricia A. Castaldi, RN, BSN, MSN
Director
Practical Nursing Program
Union County College
Plainfield, New Jersey

Margarita Valdes, RN, BS, MS
Professor of Nursing
Kingwood College
Kingwood, Texas

SKILLS PERFORMANCE CHECKLISTS:

Barbara Lauritsen Christensen, RN, MS
Nurse Educator
Mid-Plains Community College
North Platte, Nebraska

Elaine Oden Kockrow, RN, MS
Formerly, Nurse Educator
Mid-Plains Community College
North Platte, Nebraska

MOSBY
An Affiliate of Elsevier

MOSBY, INC.
An Affiliate of Elsevier
11830 Westline Industrial Drive
St. Louis, Missouri 63146

Vice President, Publishing Director: Sally Schrefer
Senior Editor: Terri Wood
Senior Developmental Editor: Robin Richman
Developmental Editor: Catherine Ott
Project Manager: Gayle May

Printed in the United States of America.

International Standard Book Number: 0-323-01737-1

Preface

This study guide has been developed as a tool to assist you in evaluating your understanding of the information presented in the *Foundations of Nursing* text. In mastering this information you will be obtaining the knowledge and necessary skills that will be important to you in your nursing practice.

The objectives from each chapter are organized under topic headings. Different learning activities are identified that will assist you to meet the content objectives. Learning activities may be matching or defining terms, completing short responses, or selecting multiple choice answers.

Study hints for completion of study guide exercises:

- Read each chapter carefully and highlight or make your own notes or outline of important information.
- Review the **Key Points** presented at the end of each chapter of the *Foundations of Nursing* textbook and complete the study questions.
- Complete the study guide exercises to the best of your ability.
- Page numbers are provided with each learning activity for your reference. Do not look up the correct answers until you have completed a section. You can repeat the exercises if you need to review the information. A complete Answer Key has been provided for your instructor.
- Time and pace yourself during the completion of each section. You should spend approximately 1 minute for each multiple choice, true false and matching; and approximately 2 minutes for completion activities or short answers.

In nursing, a strong knowledge base is important, and understanding the basic concepts and principles is necessary in order to be prepared for patient care experiences.

To the Student

This Study Guide was created to assist you in achieving the objectives of each chapter in *Foundations of Nursing*, Fourth Edition, and establishing a solid base of knowledge in the fundamentals of nursing. Completing the exercises in each chapter in this guide will help to reinforce the material studied in the textbook and learned in class. Such reinforcement also helps students to be successful on the NCLEX-PN.

Study Hints for All Students

Ask Questions!

There are no stupid questions. If you do not know something or are not sure, you need to find out. Other people may be wondering the same thing but may be too shy to ask. The answer could mean life or death to your patient. That is certainly more important than feeling embarrassed about asking a question.

Chapter Objectives

At the beginning of each chapter in the textbook are objectives that you should have mastered when you finish studying that chapter. Write these objectives in your notebook, leaving a blank space after each. Fill in the answers as you find them while reading the chapter. Review to make sure your answers are correct and complete. Use these answers when you study for tests. This should also be done for separate course objectives that your instructor has listed in your class syllabus.

Key Terms

At the beginning of each chapter in the textbook are key terms that you will encounter as you read the chapter. Text page number references are provided, for easy reference and review, and the key terms are in color the first time they appear in the chapter. Phonetic pronunciations are provided for terms that students might find difficult to pronounce. The terms that were assigned simple phonetic pronunciations were selected because they are either (1) difficult medical, nursing, or scientific terms or (2) other words that may be difficult for students to pronounce. The goal is to help the student reader with limited proficiency in English to develop a greater command of the pronunciation of scientific and nonscientific English terminology. It is hoped that a more general competency in the understanding and use of medical and scientific language may result.

Key Points

Use the Key Points at the end of each chapter in the textbook to help with review for exams.

Reading Hints

When reading each chapter in the textbook, look at the subject headings to learn what each section is about. Read first for the general meaning. Then reread parts you did not understand. It may help to read those parts aloud. Carefully read the information given in each table and study each figure and its caption.

Concepts

While studying, put difficult concepts into your own words to see if you understand them. Check this understanding with another student or the instructor. Write these in your notebook.

Class Notes

When taking lecture notes in class, leave a large margin on the left side of each notebook page and write only on right-hand pages, leaving all left-hand pages blank. Look over your lecture notes soon after each class, while your memory is fresh. Fill in missing words, complete sentences and ideas, and underline key phrases, definitions, and concepts. At the top of each page, write the topic of that page. In the left margin, write the key word for that part of your notes. On the opposite left-hand page, write a summary or outline that combines material from both the textbook and the lecture. These can be your study notes for review.

Study Groups

Form a study group with some other students so you can help one another. Practice speaking and reading aloud. Ask questions about material you are not sure about. Work together to find answers.

References for Improving Study Skills

Good study skills are essential for achieving your goals in nursing. Time management, efficient use of study time, and a consistent approach to studying are all beneficial. There are various study methods for reading a textbook and for taking class notes. Some methods that have proven helpful can be found in *Saunders Student Nurse Planner: A Guide to Success in Nursing School*. This book contains helpful information on test taking and preparing for clinical experiences. It includes an example of a "time map" for planning study time and a blank form that the student can use to formulate a personal time map.

Additional Study Hints for English as a Second Language (ESL) Students

Vocabulary

If you find a nontechnical word you do not know (e.g., *drowsy*), try to guess its meaning from the sentence (e.g., *With electrolyte imbalance, the patient may feel fatigued and drowsy*). If you are not sure of the meaning, or if it seems particularly important, look it up in the dictionary.

Vocabulary Notebook

Keep a small alphabetized notebook or address book in your pocket or purse. Write down new nontechnical words you read or hear along with their meanings and pronunciations. Write each word under its initial letter so you can find it easily, as in a dictionary. For words you do not know or for words that have a different meaning in nursing, write down how they are used and sound. Look up their meanings in a dictionary or ask your instructor or first-language buddy. Then write the different meanings or usages that you have found in your book, including the nursing meaning. Continue to add new words as you discover them. For example:

primary   • of most importance; main: *the primary problem or disease*
             • the first one; elementary: *primary school*

secondary • of less importance; resulting from another problem or disease: *a secondary symptom*
             • the second one: *secondary school (in the United States, high school)*

First Language Buddy

ESL students should find a first-language buddy—another student who is a native speaker of English and who is willing to answer questions about word meanings, pronunciations, and culture. Maybe your buddy would like to learn about your language and culture as well. This could help in his or her nursing experience as well.

Contents

UNIT ONE	BASIC NURSING CONCEPTS	
Chapter 1	The Evolution of Nursing	1
Chapter 2	Legal and Ethical Aspects of Nursing	9
Chapter 3	Communication	15
Chapter 4	Physical Assessment	21
Chapter 5	Nursing Process and Critical Thinking	29
Chapter 6	Documentation	35
Chapter 7	Cultural and Ethnic Considerations	41
Chapter 8	Life Span Development	45
Chapter 9	Loss, Grief, Dying, and Death	53

UNIT TWO	BASIC NURSING SKILLS	
Chapter 10	Admission, Transfer, and Discharge	59
Chapter 11	Vital Signs	65
Chapter 12	Medical/Surgical Asepsis and Infection Control	73
Chapter 13	Safety	81
Chapter 14	Body Mechanics and Patient Mobility	89
Chapter 15	Pain Control, Comfort, Rest, and Sleep	95
Chapter 16	Complementary and Alternative Therapies	103
Chapter 17	Hygiene and Care of the Patient's Environment	109
Chapter 18	Specimen Collection and Diagnostic Examination	117
Chapter 19	Selected Nursing Skills	125

UNIT THREE	BASIC NURSING INTERVENTIONS	
Chapter 20	Basic Nutrition and Nutritional Therapy	139
Chapter 21	Fluids and Electrolytes	153
Chapter 22	Mathematics Review and Medication Administration	161
Chapter 23	Emergency First Aid Nursing	175

UNIT FOUR	MATERNAL AND NEONATAL NURSING	
Chapter 24	Health Promotion and Pregnancy	183
Chapter 25	Labor and Delivery	191
Chapter 26	Care of the Mother and Newborn	199
Chapter 27	Care of the High-Risk Mother and Newborn	207

UNIT FIVE	PEDIATRIC NURSING	
Chapter 28	Health Promotion for the Infant, Child, and Adolescent	215
Chapter 29	Basic Pediatric Nursing Care	219
Chapter 30	Care of the Child with a Physical Disorder	227
Chapter 31	Care of the Child with a Mental or Cognitive Disorder	243

UNIT SIX   **GERONTOLOGIC NURSING**
Chapter 32   Health Promotion and Care of the Older Adult 249

UNIT SEVEN   **PSYCHIATRIC MENTAL HEALTH NURSING**
Chapter 33   Basic Concepts of Mental Health 259
Chapter 34   Care of the Patient with a Psychiatric Disorder 265
Chapter 35   Care of the Patient with an Addictive Personality 273

UNIT EIGHT   **COMMUNITY HEALTH NURSING**
Chapter 36   Home Health Nursing 281
Chapter 37   Long-Term Care 287
Chapter 38   Rehabilitation Nursing 293
Chapter 39   Hospice Care 299

UNIT NINE   **FROM GRADUATE TO PROFESSIONAL**
Chapter 40   Professional Roles and Leadership 303

                  Skills Performance Checklists 309

CHAPTER 1

Student Name _____

The Evolution of Nursing

Answer Key: Textbook page references are provided as a guide for answering these questions. A complete answer key was provided for your instructor.

TERMS

Objective

- Define the key terms as listed.

Match the terms in Column A with the appropriate definition or description in Column B.

	Column A		Column B
(7)	1. _____ Accreditation	a.	The diagnosis, treatment, and prevention of disease and the maintenance of good health
(6)	2. _____ Certification	b.	An approach to care that considers all the factors
(2)	3. _____ Health	c.	The process by which an individual's physical, emotional, intellectual, or social functioning can be diminished
(2)	4. _____ Holistic	d.	The granting of permission by a competent authority, usually government agency, which allows an individual or organization to carry out activities which would otherwise be considered illegal
(1)	5. _____ Illness		
(4)	6. _____ Licensure		
(2)	7. _____ Medicine	e.	A dynamic state of health progressing towards a higher level of functioning and optimal balance between the internal and external environments
(10)	8. _____ Wellness		
		f.	The absence of disease or other abnormal conditions; a state of mental, physical, and social well-being
		g.	The granting of recognition for an achieved competency in a specific area of nursing
		h.	The process by which a program voluntarily seeks a review by a given organization to determine whether the program meets the pre-established criteria of that organization

HISTORY OF NURSING

Objectives

- Describe the evolution of nursing and nursing education from early civilization to the 20th century.
- Identify the major leaders of nursing history in America.

(1)   9.   Nursing evolves along with changes in:

(1)   10.   In early civilization, care of the sick was primarily provided by:

(2)   11.   As far back as Ancient Egypt, there was evidence of medical treatment which included:

(2)   12.   Medicine progressed from the initial belief that illness was caused by:

(2)   13.   Discuss how monastic factors influenced the practice of nursing.

(3)   14.   What factors influenced the evolution of nursing from occupation to profession?

(4)   15.   Identify the six ways in which the "Nightingale Nurses" improved patient care and advanced the practice of nursing.

(5)   16.   Describe the effect that World War I and World War II had on nursing.

Student Name_____

(4)   17. Identify the major events that led to the development of the current nursing education programs.

Multiple Choice

(2)   18. Hippocrates is credited with development of:
1. a public system of health care.
2. a public system of safety.
3. a holistic approach to patient care.
4. early guidelines for health care.

(2)   19. Phoebe, one of the first deaconesses, was known for providing:
1. the first free hospital in Rome.
2. care to the poor and sick in their homes.
3. care for prisoners
4. care for those who were mentally ill.

(3)   20. Florence Nightingale applied the principles of nursing she learned in Germany to care of soldiers during the:
1. Civil War.
2. Spanish American War.
3. Great Plague.
4. Crimean War.

(5)   21. Which of the following individuals is credited as the first nursing theorist?
1. Mary Ann Ball
2. Clara Barton
3. Lavinia Dock
4. Florence Nightingale

(5)   22. Which of the following individuals is credited with the development and establishment of the Red Cross?
1. Dorothea Dix
2. Florence Nightingale
3. Clara Barton
4. Lavinia Dock

(5)   23. Which of the following individuals crusaded for elevation of standards of care for the mentally ill?
1. Dorothea Dix
2. Mary Ann Ball
3. Clara Barton
4. Florence Nightingale

24. Match the nursing theorists in Column A with a theory concept in Column B.

<table>
<tr><td colspan="2" align="center">**Column A**</td><td colspan="2" align="center">**Column B**</td></tr>
<tr><td>(15)</td><td>_____ Nightingale</td><td>a.</td><td>Health is a continual, open process rather than a state of well-being or absence of disease.</td></tr>
<tr><td>(15)</td><td>_____ Orem</td><td>b.</td><td>Nursing care becomes necessary when the patient is unable to fulfill biologic, psycho-logic, developmental, or social needs.</td></tr>
<tr><td>(15)</td><td>_____ Roy</td><td>c.</td><td>Caring is central to the essence of nursing.</td></tr>
<tr><td>(15)</td><td>_____ Leininger</td><td>d.</td><td>Adaptation model based on physiologic, psychologic, sociologic, and dependence-independence adaptive modes.</td></tr>
<tr><td>(15)</td><td>_____ Benner and Wrubel</td><td>e.</td><td>Patient's environment is arranged to facilitate the body's reparative processes.</td></tr>
<tr><td>(15)</td><td>_____ Parse</td><td>f.</td><td>Caring is the central and unifying domain for nursing knowledge and practice.</td></tr>
</table>

(22) 25. List the four major concepts that are the basis for nursing theories and models.

NURSING ORGANIZATIONS

Objectives

- Identify the major organizations in nursing.
- Define the four purposes of NAPNES and NFLPN.

(7) 26. Identify the role of the NLN in nursing education.

(6) 27. List the purposes of NAPNES AND NFLPN.

Student Name_____

PRACTICAL NURSING

Objectives

- List the major developments of practical/vocational nursing.
- Define practical/vocational nursing.
- Describe the purpose, role, and responsibilities of the practical/vocational nurse.

(8)   28. Identify the major development or event that occurred in the given year and give a brief description of the change that it brought about in practical/vocational nursing.

        a.   1892

        b.   1917

        c.   1941

        d.   1949

        e.   1957

        f.   1996

(15)   29. The definition that is adapted from NAPNES defines practical/vocational nursing as:

(16)   30. Discuss the role and responsibilities of the practical/vocational nurse in today's health care system.

Multiple Choice

(16)   31. The duties and responsibilities of the LPN/LVN are determined by the:
1. National League of Nursing.
2. American Nurses Association.
3. Vocational Nursing Program.
4. State Board of Nursing.

(16)   32. The content areas for the NCLEX-PN are determined by the:
1. National League of Nursing.
2. Council of State Boards of Nursing.
3. American Nurses Association.
4. Vocational Nursing Program.

HEALTH CARE DELIVERY

Objectives

- Identify the components of the health care system.
- Identify the participants of the health care system.
- Describe the complex factors involved in the delivery of patient care.

(11)   33. Identify the participants in the health care delivery system and their roles and responsibilities.

(12)   34. Identify three economic factors that influence contemporary health care delivery.

(12)   35. Provide a brief description of the following:

Malpractice insurance _____

Cross-training _____

Case management _____

(13)   36. What is the purpose of the Patient's Bill of Rights?

Student Name_____

Multiple Choice

(10) 37. Utilizing Maslow's Hierarchy of Needs, the nurse gives priority to which of the following problems of the patient?
1. loneliness
2. inability to eat
3. anxiety
4. safety

(10) 38. Utilizing Maslow's Hierarchy of Needs, which of the following needs is basic and should be addressed first?
1. safety and security
2. self-actualization
3. physiological
4. love and belonging

(12) 39. Social factors that affect health and illness are:
1. abortion, smoking, and technology.
2. health care insurance, advanced technology, and abortion.
3. patients' rights, smoking, and technology.
4. alcoholism, personal financial hardship, and social pressure.

CHAPTER 2

Student Name _____

Legal and Ethical Aspects of Nursing

Answer Key: Textbook page references are provided as a guide for answering these questions. A complete answer key was provided for your instructor.

TERMS

Objective

- Define the key terms as listed.

Match the terms in Column A with the appropriate definition or description in Column B.

Column A		Column B
(21) 1. _____ Advocate		a. Out-of-court statements made by a witness under oath
(20) 2. _____ Deposition		b. A person's agreement to allow a particular treatment to be performed based on knowledge of the facts.
(26) 3. _____ Ethical dilemmas		c. The commission or omission of an act that a reasonably prudent person would have done in a similar situation that leads to harm of another person.
(23) 4. _____ Informed consent		
(19) 5. _____ Laws		d. Defined acts that are permitted or prohibited from being performed
(22) 6. _____ Negligence		e. Rules and regulations that prescribe how individuals should act in society
(21) 7. _____ Standards of care		f. Personal beliefs about the worth of an object, idea, custom, or attitude
(25) 8. _____ Values		g. The decision based on guilt or innocence of a defendant
(26) 9. _____ Values clarification		h. Situations that do not have a clear right or wrong answer
(20) 10. _____ Verdict		i. One who will defend or plead a cause on behalf of another
		j. The process of self-evaluation by which an individual gains insight into personally held values.

LEGAL PROCESS

Objective

- Summarize the structure and function of the legal system.

(19)   11.   The two basic categories of law are:

(19)   12.   What is the difference between statutory and common law?

(20)   13.   Identify the steps in the legal process for a civil litigation.

Multiple Choice

(20)   14.   The function of criminal law is to:
   1. make the aggrieved person whole.
   2. restore the person to where he or she was.
   3. punish and prevent further crime.
   4. establish fault.

(20)   15.   The function of civil law is to:
   1. establish fault.
   2. make the aggrieved person whole.
   3. punish and prevent further crime.
   4. prevent an appeal.

(20)   16.   The individual who files the complaint in a civil litigation is referred to as the:
   1. defendant.
   2. respondent.
   3. plaintiff.
   4. prosecutor.

(20)   17.   In a criminal case the conduct or issue in question is considered to be a crime against the:
   1. court.
   2. respondent.
   3. plaintiff.
   4. society.

LEGAL RELATIONSHIPS

Objective

- Discuss the legal relationship existing between the nurse and the patient.

Student Name _____

(20)   18.   Discuss the concept of accountability and the legal relationship.

(21)   19.   Discuss areas in which the nursing staff failed to follow standards of care in the case *Darling* v. *Charleston Community Memorial Hospital.*

Multiple Choice

(21)   20.   It can be said that a nurse safeguards the nurse-patient relationship when he or she acts:
   1.   as a clinical nurse specialist with years of experience.
   2.   as an experienced nurse in a specialty area.
   3.   as other nurses with similar education and experience and in similar situations.
   4.   in accordance with the law.

REGULATION OF PRACTICE

Objectives

   • Explain the importance of maintaining standards of care.
   • Give examples of ways the nursing profession is regulated.

(21)   21.   What are the purposes of the standards of care?

(21)   22.   Evidence of nursing standards includes:

(21)   23.   How is nursing practice regulated by Nurse Practice Acts and professional organizations?

LEGAL ISSUES

Objectives

- Explain nursing malpractice.
- Give examples of ways the licensed practical/vocational nurse can avoid being involved in a lawsuit.
- Give examples of legal issues in health care.

(22)   24. Briefly define the following elements needed to establish malpractice:

Duty _____

Breach of duty _____

Harm _____

Proximate cause _____

(25)   25. Identify general ways that nurses can avoid being in lawsuits.

(22)   26. Describe the nurse's role and responsibilities in relation to the following:

Confidentiality _____

Invasion of privacy _____

Reporting of abuse _____

Multiple Choice

(22)   27. The nurse who uses unnecessary restraints on a patient may be charged with:
1. assault.
2. battery.
3. slander.
4. defamation.

(25)   28. When providing first aid in an emergency situation out side a medical facility, it is important for the nurse to have knowledge of the:
1. Nurse Practice Act.
2. Patient's Bill of Rights.
3. Good Samaritan Act.
4. standards of care.

Student Name _____

ETHICAL PRINCIPLES

Objectives

- Summarize how culture affects an individual's beliefs, morals, and values.
- Identify how values affect decision-making.

(25)   29.   The science of ethics involves the study of:

(25)   30.   Discuss how values and beliefs are developed and how they affect behavior and decision-making.

ETHICAL PRACTICE

Objectives

- Explain the meaning of a code of ethics.
- Differentiate between a legal duty and an ethical duty.
- Distinguish between ethical and unethical behavior.
- Explain the nurse's role in reporting unethical behavior.

(26)   31.   A code of ethics serves to:

(28)   32.   Indicate whether each of the following refers to a legal or ethical duty:

The nurse failed to perform in a reasonable and prudent manner. _____

The nurse failed to give the medication to the patient before he was discharged.

_____

The nurse assigned to care for an AIDS patient requested to change patients with another

nurse on the unit. _____

(27)   33.   Describe the difference between ethical and unethical behavior.

(26)   34.   List in order of priority the nursing actions to be implemented in reporting unethical behavior.

Multiple Choice

(26)   35.   The nurse demonstrates sensitivity to the cultural values and beliefs of individuals in the clinical setting by:
1.   following legal guidelines.
2.   being friendly to the patient.
3.   maintaining agency routines.
4.   individualizing patient treatment.

ETHICAL ISSUES

Objective

- Give examples of ethical issues common in health care.

(27)   36.   Discuss the following ethical issues in health care:

Right to refuse treatment

"Do not resuscitate" orders

Refusal to treat

CHAPTER 3

Communication

TERMS

Objective

- Define the key terms listed.

Match the terms in Column A with the appropriate definition or description in Column B.

	Column A		Column B
(42)	1. _____ Altered cognition	a.	Sitting with arms on chest and crossed legs
(32)	2. _____ Closed posture	b.	Inability to receive and process sent information
(30)	3. _____ Communication	c.	Sending and receiving messages
(31)	4. _____ Connotative meaning	d.	Reflects individual's perception or interpretation
(31)	5. _____ Denotative meaning	e.	Refers to a commonly accepted definition of a particular word
(46)	6. _____ Expressive aphasia	f.	Inability to send the desired message
(36)	7. _____ Focusing	g.	Used when more specific information is needed to accurately understand the patient's message
(31)	8. _____ Jargon	h.	Brief verbal comments
(36)	9. _____ Minimal encouragement	i.	Assists the patient with seeing that his or her ideas and thoughts are important in making decisions
(36)	10. _____ Reflecting	j.	Terminology unique to an individual in a specific setting

OVERVIEW

Objective

- Recognize that communication is inherent in every nurse-patient interaction.

(31)   11.   What is the goal of communication between the nurse and patient?

Multiple Choice

(30)   12.   The night nurse when giving report during shift change should be aware that a patient may hear the information being exchanged. The patient hearing the information would be referred to as the:
1. receiver.
2. sender.
3. unintended receiver.
4. communicator.

(31)   13.   In a nurse-patient relationship, when the nurse is communicating with the patient, the communication that is least effective is referred to as:
1. two-way communication.
2. one-way communication.
3. nonverbal communication.
4. open-ended communication.

TYPES OF COMMUNICATION

Objectives

- Discuss the concepts of verbal and nonverbal communication.
- Discuss the impact of nonverbal communication.
- Recognize assertive communication as the most appropriate communication style.

(31)   14.   Identify the types of verbal and nonverbal communication.

(32)   15.   Explain why consistency between verbal and nonverbal communication is important.

Student Name_____

(32) 16. Compare the characteristics of the following styles of communication:

Assertive	Aggressive	Unassertive

Multiple Choice

(31) 17. An example of nonverbal communication is:
1. moaning.
2. crying.
3. grimacing.
4. writing.

(31) 18. An example of verbal communication is:
1. writing.
2. grimacing.
3. smiling.
4. frowning.

(32) 19. Nonverbal communication involves the use of cues. Which of the following is an example of a nonverbal cue?
1. symbols
2. written words
3. reading
4. physical appearance

THERAPEUTIC COMMUNICATION

Objectives

- Use various therapeutic communication techniques.
- Recognize trust as the foundation for all effective interaction.

(33)   20. Discuss tips for building rapport with the patient.

(37)   21. Provide examples of the following therapeutic communication techniques:

Closed questioning _____

Stating observations _____

Offering information _____

Multiple Choice

(36)   22. The patient stated "I am worried and don't know what to expect after my biopsy." The nurse's reply "Are you feeling anxious about the results of your biopsy?" is an example of which of the following therapeutic communication techniques?
   1. reflection
   2. clarification
   3. restatement
   4. paraphrasing

(34)   23. The nurse is aware that providing an opportunity for receiving feedback from the patient is a way of maintaining therapeutic communication. This is an example of which of the following therapeutic communication techniques?
   1. active listening
   2. therapeutic silence
   3. minimal exchange
   4. conveying acceptance

(36)   24. The patient will be discharged from the hospital tomorrow. During the discharge teaching, the patient states, "I don't know how I will be able to care for myself after I leave the hospital." The nurse responds, "You don't know how you will take care of yourself when you leave the hospital?" This is an example of the technique of:
   1. restating.
   2. reflection.
   3. paraphrasing.
   4. summarizing.

(36)   25. In completing the patient's history, the nurse asks the patient the following information: "What type of surgeries have you had in the past?" This is an example of which of the following therapeutic communication techniques?
   1. clarifying
   2. paraphrasing
   3. restating
   4. open-ended questioning

Student Name _____

FACTORS THAT AFFECT COMMUNICATION

Objectives

- Identify various factors that can affect communication.
- Discuss potential barriers to communication.

(39)   26.   Identify the factors that may affect communication and provide an example of each.

(43)   27.   For each of the following blocks to communication, provide an example of a response that should be avoided by the nurse:

Giving advice _____

Defensiveness _____

Value judgment _____

Multiple Choice

(42)   28.   When communicating with an older adult the nurse is aware that it is important to:
1.   speak loudly.
2.   allow time for processing information.
3.   provide a dark quiet environment.
4.   avoid hearing the patient's stories.

COMMUNICATION IN SPECIAL SITUATIONS

Objectives

- Apply the nursing process to patients with impaired verbal communication.
- Apply therapeutic communication techniques to patients with special communication needs.

(44)   29.   Identify at least five nursing interventions for a client with impaired communication.

(46)   30. A 58-year-old male patient was admitted to the medical-surgical unit with diagnosis of left-sided CVA (stroke). During the admission process, the nurse observed that the patient's speech was unclear and his words were slurred. The nurse also observed that when the patient was asked a question that could be answered with a yes or no response, he could answer the question by moving his head to imply yes or no. Apply the nursing process to the given situation.

Identify problems observed by the nurse during the admission process.

Write a nursing diagnosis based on the identified problems.

Write a realistic goal for the nursing diagnosis.

Identify at least two nursing actions can be implemented.

Write a statement that reflects the evaluation of the outcome.

Multiple Choice

(46)   31. When communicating with a patient who has expressive aphasia, the nurse is aware that it is important to:
1. ask open-ended questions.
2. ask questions that can be answered with a yes or no.
3. refer to the family members for information.
4. allow a short time for the patient to respond.

CHAPTER 4

Student Name _____

Physical Assessment

Answer Key: Textbook page references are provided as a guide for answering these questions. A complete answer key was provided for your instructor.

TERMS

Objective

- Define the key terms as listed.

Match the terms in Column A with the appropriate definition or description in Column B.

	Column A		Column B
(50)	1. _____ Acute	a.	Abnormal "swishing" sound heard over arteries
(67)	2. _____ Borborygmi	b.	The elasticity of the skin
(63)	3. _____ Bruit	c.	Begins abruptly with intense signs and symptoms
(50)	4. _____ Chronic	d.	High-pitched, loud, rushing bowel sound
(55)	5. _____ Dullness	e.	Develops slowly and persists over a long period of time
(50)	6. _____ Erythema	f.	Fluid, cells, or other debris that have been slowly discharged
(49)	7. _____ Etiology	g.	Vibrating sensation along the arteries that can be palpated
(48)	8. _____ Exudate	h.	A thudlike sound heard with percussion
(61)	9. _____ Focused assessment	i.	Examination fails to reveal evidence of structural or physiological abnormalities
(50)	10. _____ Functional disease	j.	Refers to cause of disease
(63)	11. _____ Thrill	k.	High-pitched, drumlike sound heard with percussion
(62)	12. _____ Turgor	l.	Sibilant or sonorous sound produced by fluid in the bronchioles and alveoli
(55)	13. _____ Tympany	m.	Attention is concentrated on a specific area of the body
(64)	14. _____ Wheeze	n.	Redness; result of dilation and congestion of superficial capillaries

DISEASE AND DIAGNOSIS

Objectives

- Discuss the difference between a sign and a symptom.
- Compare and contrast the origins of disease.
- List the four major risk categories for development of disease.
- Discuss frequently noted signs and symptoms of disease conditions.
- List the cardinal signs of inflammation and infection.

(48) 15. Identify the difference between a sign and a symptom.

(48) 16. Identify whether each of the following is a sign or a symptom:

Headache _____

Nausea _____

Anxiety _____

Vomiting_____

Drainage _____

(49) 17. Identify at least five possible etiologies of disease.

(50) 18. The four major risk categories for the development of disease are:

(50) 19. The cardinal signs of infection and inflammation are:

Student Name_____

Multiple Choice

(49)   20.   Diseases that are hereditary:
1.   have unknown etiology.
2.   appear at birth.
3.   are transmitted from parent to children.
4.   are a result of an infection.

(49)   21.   Autoimmune diseases:
1.   appear at birth.
2.   are transmitted from parent to children.
3.   have unknown etiology.
4.   are a result of infection.

(49)   22.   Deficiency diseases are a result of:
1.   lack of nutrients.
2.   abnormal growth of tissue.
3.   exposure to microorganisms.
4.   harmful substances.

(50)   23.   The risk factor that can lead to the development of coronary artery disease is:
1.   osteoporosis.
2.   cancer.
3.   stress.
4.   sunbathing.

(50)   24.   A lifestyle risk that can lead to the development of lung disease is:
1.   air pollution.
2.   asbestos.
3.   smoking.
4.   malnutrition.

(51)   25.   While obtaining the vital signs, the nurse observed that the patient was sweating profusely. The term used to describe this sign is:
1.   diaphoresis.
2.   cyanosis.
3.   ecchymosis.
4.   pruritus.

(51)   26.   When assessing the patient's skin color, the nurse noted that the skin and mucous membranes had a bluish discoloration. The term used to describe this sign is:
1.   jaundice.
2.   pallor.
3.   cyanosis.
4.   ecchymosis.

(51)   27.   While transferring the patient from the stretcher to the bed, the nurse observed that the patient was experiencing difficulty breathing. The term used to describe this sign is:
1.   orthopnea.
2.   dyspnea.
3.   tachypnea.
4.   asthenia.

(51)   28. The patient's oral temperature is 101.2° F. The term used to describe this sign is:
1. edema.
2. febrile.
3. pruritus.
4. jaundice.

(51)   29. The patient informed the nurse that she was not hungry and had been experiencing loss of appetite for several days. The term used to describe this symptom is:
1. lethargy.
2. dyspnea.
3. anorexia.
4. erythema.

(51)   30. When assessing the older adult the nurse is aware that slumping, irritability, or sighing can indicate that the patient is exhibiting signs related to the symptom of:
1. dyspnea.
2. fatigue.
3. orthopnea.
4. erythema.

(49)   31. Which of the following is an example of objective data?
1. pulse
2. nausea
3. pain
4. fear

(48)   32. Which of the following is an example of subjective data?
1. blood pressure
2. edema
3. pain
4. erythema

MEDICAL EXAMINATION

Objectives

- Describe the nursing responsibilities when assisting a physician with the physical examination.
- List equipment and supplies necessary for the physical examination/assessment.

(52)   33. When assisting the physician with the physical examination, the nurse is responsible for:

(53)   34. For the following parts of the examination, identify the position(s) of the patient:

Head and neck _____

Thorax _____

Abdomen _____

Female genitalia _____

Musculoskeletal system _____

(61)   35.   Identify the equipment needed to assess or examine the following:

Vital signs _____

Lung sounds _____

Reflexes _____

(52)   36.   Discuss the nursing responsibilities related to the psychological preparation of the patient for a physical examination.

NURSING ASSESSMENT

Objectives

- Explain the necessary skills for the physical examination/nursing assessment.
- Discuss the nurse-patient interview.
- List the essentials for a patient's health history.
- Discuss the sequence of steps when performing a nursing assessment.
- Explain ways to develop cultural sensitivity.

(58)   37.   Provide examples of questions that may be asked by the nurse to obtain information during a review of systems.

Respiratory _____

Endocrine _____

Gastrointestinal _____

(63)   38.   When preparing to check the patient's pupillary reflexes, the nurse must first:

(55)   39.   Identify the skills used in the physical/nursing assessment and the purpose of each one.

(56)   40.   Identify five elements that can enhance the nurse-patient interview.

(56)   41.   The objectives of the nursing health history are:

(57)   42.   List the essential information obtained in a health history that will assist the nurse in developing the patient's plan of care.

(59)   43.   Identify ways that the nurse may develop cultural sensitivity in relation to the physical examination.

(70)   44.   What does each letter represent in the mnemonic device for assessing patients?

A   _____

B   _____

C   _____

In   _____

Student Name_____

Out _____

P _____

S _____

Multiple Choice

(57)   45.   The nurse utilizes the PQRST method for obtaining the most information about the patient's present health concerns. The P in the PQRST method refers to the:
1. quality of the concern.
2. cause of the concern.
3. severity of the concern.
4. beginning of the concern.

(55)   46.   The most frequently used skill in the physical nursing assessment is:
1. inspection.
2. palpation.
3. percussion.
4. auscultation.

ASSESSMENT FINDINGS

Objective

- Discuss normal assessment findings in the head-to-toe assessment.

(62)   47.   Identify whether the following findings are expected or unexpected.

Decreased skin turgor_____

Fruity breath_____

Pupils round and reactive to light _____

Barrel chest_____

Two-second capillary refill _____

Adventitious breath sounds _____

No abdominal sounds _____

Bilateral, palpable pedal pulses _____

DOCUMENTATION

Objective

- Describe documentation of the physical examination/nursing assessment.

(69)   48.   How are physical assessment results usually documented?

What is important for the nurse to do when documenting findings?

CHAPTER 5

Nursing Process and Critical Thinking

Student Name _____

Answer Key: Textbook page references are provided as a guide for answering these questions. A complete answer key was provided for your instructor.

TERMS

Objective

- Define the key terms as listed.

Match the terms in Column A with the appropriate definition or description in Column B.

	Column A		Column B
(75)	1. _____ Biographical data	a.	A clinical judgment that a problem may develop
(83)	2. _____ Case management	b.	Used to identify a cluster of actual or risk nursing diagnoses
(83)	3. _____ Critical pathway	c.	"Readiness for Enhanced Nutrition"
(74)	4. _____ Cue	d.	Cues/signs/symptoms that furnish evidence that the problem exists
(77)	5. _____ Defining characteristics	e.	Provides pertinent information about facts or events in a person's life
(75)	6. _____ NANDA	f.	A statement that describes a specific measurable behavior
(79)	7. _____ Outcome	g.	When an expected outcome is not reached.
(75)	8. _____ Problem	h.	Assignment of a health care provider to an individual patient
(77)	9. _____ Risk nursing diagnosis	i.	A multidisciplinary plan for clinical interventions
(78)	10. _____ Syndrome nursing diagnosis	j.	Subjective or objective data
		k.	North American Nursing Diagnosis Association
(84)	11. _____ Variance	l.	Any health care condition that requires intervention
(78)	12. _____ Wellness nursing diagnosis		

PHASES OF THE NURSING PROCESS

Objectives

- Explain the use of each of the five phases of the nursing process.
- List the elements of each of the five phases of the nursing process.

(73)   13. The five phases of the nursing process are:

Multiple Choice

(73)   14. The nursing process:
1. provides the patient with quality care.
2. focuses on a specific patient-related problem.
3. provides a framework for the practice of nursing.
4. ensures positive outcomes.

(73)   15. The patient's information and data are collected during the:
1. assessment phase.
2. planning phase.
3. implementation phase.
4. evaluation phase.

(75)   16. During which phase of the nursing process does the nurse identify the health problems?
1. assessment
2. diagnosis
3. planning
4. implementation

(78)   17. The nurse sets priorities for nursing intervention in the:
1. assessment phase.
2. diagnosis phase.
3. planning phase.
4. implementation phase

(78)   18. The nurse establishes the patient goals and outcomes during the:
1. assessment phase.
2. planning phase.
3. implementation phase.
4. evaluation phase.

(82)   19. The nurse instructs the patient on the use of her inhaler. During which phase of the nursing process does this take place?
1. diagnosis
2. planning
3. implementation
4. evaluation

(82)   20. Documentation is a vital component of:
1. assessment.
2. diagnosis.
3. implementation.
4. evaluation.

ASSESSMENT

Objective

- Describe the establishment of the database.

(75)   21. What sources are used to obtain information for the patient database?

Multiple Choice

(75)   22. After collecting and validating the data, the nurse organizes and clusters the data. Data clustering refers to:
1. the evaluation of the patient data.
2. focusing on the patient's problems.
3. the grouping of related cues.
4. the analysis of related outcomes.

DIAGNOSIS

Objectives

- Discuss the steps used to formulate a nursing diagnosis.
- Differentiate among types of health problems.

(76)   23. Write a possible nursing diagnosis based upon the following situation:

A 52-year-old client is admitted after episodes of severe vomiting.

Multiple Choice

(75)   24. The nursing diagnosis is defined as:
1. the identification of a disease or condition that involves problems with structures.
2. problems that nurses cannot prescribe a treatment for.
3. A clinical judgment about individual, group, or community responses to actual or potential health problems.
4. problems that are identified as a result of the planning phase.

(75)   25. At the completion of the nursing assessment phase, the nursing diagnosis statement is formulated and a "possible diagnosis" statement may be written by the nurse. The "possible diagnosis" statement is written when the:
1.   actual or risk factors are predicted to be present in a circumstance.
2.   database does not provide sufficient evidence that an actual problem exists.
3.   database provides evidence of an actual problem.
4.   cues obtained from a nursing assessment indicate a problem exists.

(78)   26. Based on the definition of a collaborative problem, which of the following problems would be an example?
1.   pain
2.   anxiety
3.   coping
4.   edema

PLANNING

Objectives

- Describe the development of patient-centered outcomes.
- Discuss the creation of nursing orders.

(79)   27. Identify Maslow's Hierarchy of Needs beginning with the ones that are given highest priority in patient care situations.

(79)   28. Patient-centered outcomes should be statements that are:

(80)   29. What is included in a nursing order?

(80)   30. Write an example of a nursing order.

Multiple Choice

(80)   31.   A nursing order is created to provide:
1. specific written instructions for all caregivers.
2. a general statement that conveys information.
3. a statement providing general information for nursing interventions.
4. information for the formulation of a care plan.

EVALUATION

Objective

- Explain the evaluation of a nursing care plan.

(82)   32.   Describe the steps in the evaluation of the nursing care plan.

CARE PLANS AND CLINICAL PATHWAYS

Objectives

- Demonstrate the nursing process by writing a nursing care plan.
- Describe the use of clinical pathways in managed care.

(83)   33.   Identify the purpose and advantages of clinical pathways.

(81)   34.   Write a nursing care plan for the following patient situation:

Ms. M., 48 years of age, is admitted to the medical-surgical unit after an abdominal hysterectomy. Her vital signs are stable. The IV in her left forearm is patent, without swelling or tenderness. The dressings are dry and intact. Ms. M. has a Foley catheter in place that is draining clear, yellow urine. Ms. M. was just transferred from the surgical recovery unit. Ms. M. is expressing severe pain.

GROUPS

Objective

- Explain the activities of NANDA, NIC, and NOC.

(82)   35.   Identify the general activities of NANDA, NIC, and NOC.

CRITICAL THINKING

Objective

- Discuss critical thinking.

(85)   36.   Provide specific examples of how critical thinking is applied in clinical nursing situations.

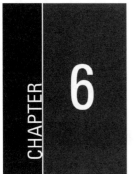

CHAPTER 6

Student Name _____

Documentation

Answer Key: Textbook page references are provided as a guide for answering these questions. A complete answer key was provided for your instructor.

TERMS

Objective

- Define the key terms as listed.

Match the terms in Column A with the appropriate definition or description in Column B.

	Column A		Column B
(90)	1. _____ Auditors	a.	Written information contained in the patient records
(89)	2. _____ Chart	b.	Persons appointed to examine patients' charts and health records to assess quality of care
(89)	3. _____ Charting	c.	A legal record used to meet the many demands of the health systems
(90)	4. _____ Database	d.	Audit that evaluates care and services provided in health care
(99)	5. _____ Kardex/Rand	e.	An appraisal of individual nursing conduct by equals
(90)	6. _____ Narrative charting	f.	Form used by nurses to record their observations, care given, and the patient's response
(90)	7. _____ Nursing note	g.	A system used to consolidate patient orders and care needs in a centralized, concise way
(90)	8. _____ Peer review	h.	A summary form of charting that should include the basic needs of the patient, whether someone was contacted, care and treatment provided, and the patient's response
(90)	9. _____ Quality assurance/ assessment/ improvement	i.	Documentation of care
(91)	10. _____ SOAPE	j.	Subjective/objective assessment, plan, evaluation; in this more compact form, the care given or action taken is included in the plan notations

PURPOSES

Objectives

- List the five purposes for written patient records.
- Explain the relationship of the nursing care plan to care documentation and patient care reimbursement.

(89)   11.   The five basic purposes of written patient records are:

(102)   12.   Identify how home health care documentation relates to reimbursement.

Multiple Choice

(90)   13.   A system that is used by Medicare for reimbursement of patient care services is:
             1.   focused medical-related grouping.
             2.   diagnosis-related group.
             3.   quality assurance/improvement.
             4.   problem-oriented diagnosis-related group.

METHODS AND FORMS

Objectives

- Describe the differences between traditional and problem-oriented medical records.
- Describe the purpose of and relationship between the Kardex and the nursing care plan.
- Describe the differences in documenting care using activities of daily living and physical assessment forms, narrative, SOAPE, and focus formats.
- Discuss the use of computers for recordkeeping and documentation in health care facilities.
- Discuss documentation and clinical pathways.

(99)   14.   What is the purpose of an incident report?

             Is the incident report included in the patient's record? _____

(99)   15.   Describe the relationship between the Kardex and the patient chart.

(103)   16.   What are the advantages and disadvantages of computer documentation?

(101)   17.   Identify the primary benefit of documenting with clinical pathways.

Multiple Choice

(92)   18.   Focus charting contains:
1.   nursing action and patient response.
2.   a description of the patient's present condition.
3.   objective and subjective assessment data.
4.   nursing diagnosis, action, and patient's response.

(96)   19.   Charting by exception:
1.   provides comprehensive nurse's notes.
2.   provides a more organized flow in the nurse's notes.
3.   decreases the length of time needed to complete the nurse's notes.
4.   summarizes the information in the nurse's notes.

(90)   20.   Traditional charting:
1.   is organized and specific to patient-related care.
2.   allows only the physicians to enter information on the progress note.
3.   allows all members of the health care team to record on the same form.
4.   utilizes a problem list in documenting patient care.

(90)   21.   What type of charting format usually requires the most time to complete?
1.   SOAP
2.   focus
3.   PIE
4.   narrative

(98)   22.   What type of charting format most reflects the nursing process?
1.   narrative
2.   traditional
3.   focus
4.   PIE

(98)   23.   What documentation is included in the "P" when using the PIE method of charting?
1.   patient response
2.   problem list
3.   assessment
4.   plan

(90)   24. The POMR is divided into which four major sections?
1.   history and physical examination, physician's orders, nurse's notes, and progress notes
2.   database, problem list, plan, and progress notes
3.   subjective data, objective data, diagnostic tests, and progress notes
4.   physician's orders, nurse's notes, lab reports, and progress notes

(90)   25. Traditional medical records:
1.   utilize a patient problem list as index for chart documenting.
2.   utilize a narrative format for documenting nurse's notes.
3.   utilize care plans for documenting in the nurses notes.
4.   emphasize the use of specific sheets for charting.

(90)   26. The problem-oriented medical record:
1.   utilizes a patient problem list as index for chart documenting.
2.   utilizes a narrative format for documenting nurses notes.
3.   utilizes care plans for documenting in the nurse's notes.
4.   emphasizes the use of specific sheets for charting.

(101)   27. The charting format most commonly used for documentation of clinical pathways is:
1.   focus charting.
2.   traditional charting.
3.   charting by exception.
4.   narrative charting.

GUIDELINES

Objectives

- Describe the basic guidelines for and mechanics of charting.
- State important legal aspects of chart ownership, access, confidentiality, and patient care documentation.

(104)   28. The essential elements of documentation are:

(98)   29. What are the basic guidelines for charting?

Student Name _____

(102)   30.   Identify the important legal aspects for the following:

Chart ownership _____

Access _____

Confidentiality _____

(101)   31.   Military time is used in most of the hospitals to document the time care is given. Convert the following civilian times to military time.

3:00 PM _____

7:30 PM _____

6:00 PM _____

midnight _____

Multiple Choice

(98)   32.   When an error is made by the nurse in charting,
1.   it is reported to the charge nurse and the nurse continues with the charting.
2.   white-out is used to correct the error and the nurse continues with the charting.
3.   the charting is started over on a new sheet.
4.   a line is drawn through the error and initialed and then the nurse continues with the charting.

(103)   33.   Confidentiality is most often maintained with use of computer charting through the:
1.   assignment of individual entry passwords.
2.   legal signature of the nurse.
3.   use of patient code names.
4.   use of assigned individual patient unit numbers.

(102)   34.   The patient can gain access to his or her records/chart:
1.   in all states.
2.   immediately upon request of the information.
3.   with a formal written request.
4.   by following established procedures of the facility or institution.

(102)   35.   Confidentiality of the patient's medical information is guaranteed by the:
1.   law.
2.   American Hospital Association.
3.   standards of care.
4.   Code of Ethics.

HEALTH CARE SITES

Objectives

- Discuss long-term health care documentation.
- Discuss home health care documentation.

(102)   36.   In relation to documentation, the Omnibus Budget Reconciliation Act (OBRA) of 1987 requires:

(101)   37.   Briefly identify how long-term care and home health care documentation are different from acute care (hospital) documentation.

CHAPTER 7

Cultural and Ethnic Considerations

Answer Key: Textbook page references are provided as a guide for answering these questions. A complete answer key was provided for your instructor.

TERMS

Objective

- Define the key terms as listed.

Match the terms in Column A with the appropriate definition or description in Column B.

	Column A		Column B
(119)	1. _____ Biomedical health belief system	a.	Nursing awareness of personal culture, beliefs, and practices of individual patients
(107)	2. _____ Culture	b.	A group of people who share biological characteristics
(108)	3. _____ Cultural competence	c.	A group of people who share common social and cultural heritage based on traditions and national origin
(108)	4. _____ Ethnicity	d.	Fixed concept about how all members of an ethnic group act or think
(108)	5. _____ Ethnic stereotype	e.	The belief that disease has specific cause, length of onset, course, and treatment
(110)	6. _____ Ethnocentrism	f.	Learned beliefs, customs, and practices shared by a group and passed to another generation
(119)	7. _____ Holistic health belief system	g.	The belief that one's own culture is superior to other cultures; the judging of other cultures by the standards of one's own culture
(108)	8. _____ Mores	h.	Treatment is designed to restore balance with physical, social, and metaphysical worlds
(108)	9. _____ Race	i.	Accepted traditional customs, moral attitudes, or manner of particular social group
(107)	10. _____ Society	j.	Made up of a broad group of people who establish particular aims, beliefs, or standards of living and conduct

CULTURE AND ETHNICITY

Objective

- Describe ways that culture affects the individual.

Multiple Choice

(107)   11. Two groups sharing primary characteristics but having different behaviors and ideas describes a(n):
1. ethnic group.
2. dominant group.
3. subculture.
4. race.

HEALTH BELIEFS AND PRACTICES

Objectives

- Explain how personal cultural beliefs and practices can affect nurse-patient and nurse-nurse relationships.
- Identify and discuss cultural variables that may influence health behaviors.

(112)   12. Describe how the following cultural variables influence health behaviors.

Family structure _____

Religious beliefs _____

Health practices _____

(121)   13. Compare and contrast two different cultural groups in relation to the following:

Time orientation _____

Dietary preferences_____

Birth rites _____

Multiple Choice

(119)   14. Which of the following statements best describes cultural influence on health beliefs?
1. Patients respond the same to healing touch.
2. All cultures value traditional medicine.
3. The response to health and illness varies among different cultures.
4. Based on cultural data, the nurse makes certain assumptions about the patient.

(118)   15. Which of the following religious groups believes that blood transfusions violate God's laws?
1. Quaker
2. Mennonite
3. Jehovah's Witnesses
4. Roman Catholics

NURSING PROCESS

Objectives

- Identify the importance of transcultural nursing.
- Explain how cultural data can be used to assist the nurse to develop therapeutic relationships with the patient.
- Discuss the use of the nursing process when caring for culturally diverse patients.

(107)   16. How does the nurse integrate transcultural nursing into practice?

(108)   17. List considerations related to cultural differences that nurses need to be aware of when caring for an older adult.

(110)   18. Identify nursing interventions that may be used to communicate with a non-English–speaking patient.

(109)   19. In order to assist the patient to meet his/her needs, the nurse wants to complete an accurate assessment. How should the nurse ask the patient about the following?

Language _____

Illness _____

Family structure _____

Dietary practices _____

Use of folk medicine _____

(120)   20. Write a nursing diagnosis that can be modified to reflect the problems of a culturally diverse patient.

Multiple Choice

(108)   21. Transcultural nursing is:
1.   nursing care that is given to a group of patients who share specific beliefs.
2.   nursing care based on a specific group's behavior and needs.
3.   the implementation of culturally appropriate nursing care.
4.   the implementation of generalized standards of care to meet needs of all patients.

(111)   22. When communicating with a patient who has a poor grasp of English, the nurse should:
1.   speak loudly.
2.   keep questions brief and simple.
3.   use sign language and get an interpreter.
4.   provide detailed directions.

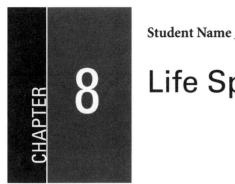

CHAPTER 8

Life Span Development

Answer Key: Textbook page references are provided as a guide for answering these questions. A complete answer key was provided for your instructor.

TERMS

Objective

- Define the key terms listed.

Match the terms in Column A with the appropriate definition or description in Column B.

		Column A		Column B
(155)	1. _____	Ageism	a.	Anything that physically or psychologically injures school children or damages school property
(128)	2. _____	Cephalocaudal	b.	An innate knowledge structure that allows a child to mentally organize ways to behave in immediate environment
(129)	3. _____	Chromosomes		
(128)	4. _____	Conception (fertilization)	c.	Increase in size of the whole or its parts
			d.	Function or gradual process of change from simple to complex
(150)	5. _____	Depression	e.	Development from head to toe
(128)	6. _____	Development	f.	Substance, agent, or process that interferes with normal prenatal development
(128)	7. _____	Growth	g.	Union of sperm and ovum
(127)	8. _____	Life expectancy	h.	A form of discrimination and prejudice against older adults
(153)	9. _____	Presbycusis	i.	Developing ovum from fertilization to blastocyst
(152)	10. _____	Presbyopia	j.	Threadlike structures in the nucleus of a cell that function in transmission of genetic information
(128)	11. _____	Proximodistal		
(134)	12. _____	Schema	k.	Center towards the outside
(147)	13. _____	School violence	l.	Disturbance characterized by feeling of sadness, despair, and hopelessness
(129)	14. _____	Teratogen	m.	Normal loss of hearing
			n.	Far-sightedness
(129)	15. _____	Zygote	o.	Average number of years an individual will probably live

FAMILY

Objectives

- Differentiate among the types of family patterns and their functions in society.
- Describe different types of stresses that commonly affect today's families.

(129)   16.   Families are composed of two or more people who are united by:

(130)   17.   List the four family patterns and describe their functions.

(129)   18.   Identify factors that have contributed to the changed/changing family.

(131)   19.   Discuss the qualities of functional families.

(132)   20.   Three common causes of family stress are:

Multiple Choice

(130)   21.   The nuclear family is:
   1.   biological parents, offspring, and grandparents.
   2.   biological parents, offspring, grandparents, aunts, and uncles.
   3.   biological parents and their offspring.
   4.   traditional family and some additional family members.

Student Name_____

(130) 22. A social contract family consists of:
1.   remarried adults and children.
2.   same-sex couple with foster or adoptive children.
3.   the family unit with adopted children.
4.   an unmarried couple living together and sharing roles and responsibilities.

GROWTH AND DEVELOPMENT

Objectives

- Describe the physical characteristics at each stage of the life cycle.
- List the psychosocial changes at the different stages of development.
- Discuss Erikson's stages of psychosocial development.
- Describe Piaget's four stages of cognitive development.

INFANCY, TODDLER, PRESCHOOL, SCHOOL AGE

Objective

- Describe the cognitive changes occurring in the early childhood period.

(132) 23. Children may be affected by stress. Identify at least five common signs of stress in children.

(133) 24. Identify the major physical and psychosocial changes that occur from infancy through school age.

	Physical Changes	**Psychosocial Changes**
Infant		
Toddler		
Preschooler		

Multiple Choice

(133)   25.   Height increases approximately _____ a month for the first 6 months of life.
1.   ½ inch
2.   1 inch
3.   2 inches
4.   3 inches

(133)   26.   By the time an infant is 1 year of age, the child will have:
1.   doubled his or her birth weight.
2.   gained 1 lb per month.
3.   tripled his or her birth weight.
4.   gained 3 lbs per month.

(133)   27.   Weight gain after 8 months is attributed to:
1.   fat and muscle.
2.   fat and bone.
3.   fat and increased fluid volume.
4.   muscle and bone.

(145)   28.   Obvious growth in the long bones and increase in height of approximately 2 inches per year for both boys and girls are physical characteristics of:
1.   preschoolers.
2.   toddlers.
3.   school-age children.
4.   adolescents.

(140)   29.   By the age of 2½ years the toddler has:
1.   complete primary dentition, 20 teeth.
2.   approximately 16 teeth present.
3.   approximately 12 teeth.
4.   approximately 30 teeth.

(136)   30.   The infant uses the senses to learn about self and environment in the:
1.   formal operational stage.
2.   preoperational stage.
3.   sensorimotor stage.
4.   concrete operational stage.

(136)   31.   The toddler gradually begins to "de-center" (becomes less egocentric and understands other points of view) in the:
1.   formal operational stage.
2.   preoperational stage.
3.   sensorimotor stage.
4.   concrete operational stage.

(136)   32.   The school-age child is able to think about abstractions and hypothetical concepts and is able to move in thought "from the real to the possible" in the:
1.   formal operational stage.
2.   preoperational stage.
3.   sensorimotor stage.
4.   concrete operational stage.

Student Name_____

(143)   33. The cognitive stage of early childhood extends from:
   1. 1–3 years of age.
   2. 2–7 years of age.
   3. 5–9 years of age.
   4. 9–12 years of age.

ADOLESCENCE

Objective

- Discuss the developmental tasks of the adolescent period.

(150)   34. Identify at least five developmental tasks of the adolescent.

Multiple Choice

(148)   35. The second major period of rapid physical growth is observed in the:
   1. school-age child.
   2. adolescent.
   3. young adult.
   4. middle adult.

YOUNG AND MIDDLE ADULTHOOD

Objectives

- List the developmental tasks for early adulthood.
- Describe the developmental tasks for middle adulthood.

(152)   36. Provide examples of the developmental tasks for the early and middle adult.

Multiple Choice

(153)   37. Generativity can best be defined as:
   1. the ability to relate one's deepest hopes and concerns to another person.
   2. the task of reorganization, reevaluation, and acceptance.
   3. accepting responsibility for and offering guidance to the next generation and adapting to physical and role changes.
   4. a time of satisfaction and pleasure.

LATE ADULTHOOD

Objectives

- Define aging.
- Discuss theories of aging.
- Describe the normal age-related changes affecting the major body systems.
- Discuss the effect of the aging process on personality, intelligence, learning, and memory.

38.   Match the theory in Column A with the appropriate definition or description in Column B.

	Column A		Column B
(156)	_____ Autoimmunity theory	a.	The aging process will be eased by maintaining roles and interests similar to those developed earlier in life.
(156)	_____ Biologic programming theory	b.	There should be a natural withdrawal of the individual from society.
(156)	_____ Disengagement theory	c.	This describes hereditary basis for aging, evidenced by the similarities in life expectancies in a particular family.
(156)	_____ Free radical theory	d.	These are highly reactive cellular components derived from unstable atoms or molecules may accelerate aging.
(156)	_____ Continuity theory	e.	This theory is supported by increased accumulation of lymphocytes and plasma cells found in normal, healthy, older persons.

(157)   39.   Describe the physical changes that occur in each of the following systems as a result of the aging process:

Sensory _____

Integumentary _____

Cardiovascular _____

Respiratory _____

Gastrointestinal _____

Genitourinary _____

Musculoskeletal _____

Neurological _____

Student Name_____

(157)   40.   What influence does the aging process have on the following?

Personality _____

Intelligence and learning _____

Memory _____

Multiple Choice

(154)   41.   Aging is best defined as a:
1. period of decline in social activities.
2. period in which senility increased.
3. normal condition of human existence that can be affected by health habits and family.
4. normal state in which changes in physiological conditions are universal and inevitable.

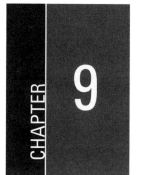

CHAPTER 9

Loss, Grief, Dying, and Death

Answer Key: Textbook page references are provided as a guide for answering these questions. A complete answer key was provided for your instructor.

TERMS

Objective

- Define the key terms as listed.

Match the terms in Column A with the appropriate definition or description in Column B.

	Column A		Column B
(175)	1. _____ Advance directives	a.	Unresolved grief or complicated mourning
(166)	2. _____ Anticipatory grief	b.	Study of death and dying
(165)	3. _____ Bereavement	c.	An illness or an abnormal condition or quality
(175)	4. _____ Durable power of attorney	d.	To expect, await, or prepare oneself for the loss of a family member or significant other
(168)	5. _____ Dysfunctional grieving	e.	A common depressed reaction to the death of a loved one
(175)	6. _____ Euthanasia	f.	Condition being subject to death
(163)	7. _____ Grief	g.	A pattern of physical or emotional responses to bereavement, separation, or loss
(165)	8. _____ Morbidity	h.	A signed and witnessed document providing specific instructions for health care treatments in the that a person is unable to make those decisions
(163)	9. _____ Mortality	i.	An action deliberately taken with the purpose of shortening life to end suffering or carry out the wishes of a terminally ill patient
(167)	10. _____ Thanatology	j.	A signed and dated document that must be notarized and which gives one or more individuals (proxies) the ability to make decision on behalf of a person

GRIEF AND LOSS

Objectives

- Explain how the concept of loss affects the grief reaction.
- Recognize the five aspects of human functioning and how each interacts with the others during the grieving/dying process.

(164)   11.   Briefly describe the concepts of loss and grief.

(164)   12.   Identify at least seven factors that influence the experience of loss.

(169)   13.   Discuss how physical and social aspects of human functioning influence the grieving process.

Multiple Choice

(164)   14.   Maturational loss is best defined as:
1. a loss occurring suddenly in response to a specific external event.
2. any significant loss that requires adaptation through the grieving process.
3. a loss resulting from normal life transitions.
4. events such as the death of a loved one, divorce, breakup of a relationship, or loss of a job.

(164)   15.   Situational loss can best be defined as:
1. a loss occurring suddenly in response to a specific external event.
2. any significant loss that requires adaptation through the grieving process.
3. a loss resulting from normal life transitions.
4. events such as the death of a loved one, divorce, breakup of a relationship, or loss of a job.

Student Name_____

STAGES OF GRIEF AND DYING

Objectives
- Describe the stages of dying.
- Identify needs of the grieving patient and family.
- Discuss support for the grieving family.
- Discuss approaches to facilitate the grieving process.

(167)   16.   Identify Kubler-Ross' stage of dying in each of the following examples of patient responses:

"No, not me." _____

"I just want to live until my daughter gets married." _____

"It's not fair. I can't stand this!" _____

(169)   17.   Identify the nursing assessments and interventions for the patient/family experiencing death and grieving.

	Assessment	Interventions
Physical needs		
Emotional needs		
Spiritual needs		

(167)   18.   It is important that the nurse have knowledge and an understanding of survivors' reactions in identifying and meeting the needs of the grieving family. List and describe Martocchio's Manifestations of Grief or Survivors' Reaction.

NURSING PROCESS

Objectives

- Identify unique physical signs and symptoms of the near-death patient.
- Discuss nursing interventions for the dying patient.
- Describe techniques in assisting the dying patient to say good-bye.
- Identify how the changes in the health care system affect nursing interventions for the dying patient.
- Describe nursing responsibilities in care of the body after death.

(168)   19. Write a nursing diagnosis, patient outcome, and nursing interventions based on the following situation:

The patient lost her husband in an automobile accident a year ago. She is still experiencing insomnia and feelings of worthlessness and anger, and she continues to avoid family or social functions.

(166)   20. Provide examples of how nurses cope with grief when they deal with their dying patients.

(179)   21. Identify the changes in vital signs that occur in the patient who is near death.

(179)   22. What are the priority needs of the dying patient?

(178)   23. Provide examples of some techniques that nurses may use to assist patients to say good-bye.

Student Name_____

(181)   24. Number the following nursing actions in the order that they should be done, from first to last:

Remove all tubing and other devices. _____

Wash hands and don gloves. _____

Place patient in supine position. _____

Bathe patient as necessary. _____

Close patient's eyes and mouth if needed. _____

Allow family to view body and remain in the room. _____

SPECIAL SUPPORTIVE CARE

Objective

- List nursing interventions that may facilitate grieving in special circumstances.

(174)   25. Identify nursing interventions to facilitate grieving in the following special circumstances:

Perinatal death _____

Pediatric death _____

Geriatric death _____

Suicide _____

ISSUES RELATED TO DEATH AND DYING

Objectives

- Explain advance directives, which include the living will and durable power of attorney.
- Explain concepts of euthanasia, DNR, organ donations, fraudulent methods of treatment, and the Dying Person's Bill of Rights.

(177)   26. Provide examples of fraudulent methods of treatment that may be offered to the dying patient/family.

Multiple Choice

(175) 27. The terminally ill patient has been experiencing severe pain and has requested that the doctor assist her to end her suffering. The appropriate term used when referring to the action of ending this patient's life is:
1. euthanasia.
2. passive suicide.
3. brain death.
4. mercy killing.

(176) 28. The patient in room 318 has a DNR order. The licensed vocational nurse knows that a DNR order means:
1. withholding of nutrition.
2. ddministering pain medication.
3. not administering CPR if the patient stops breathing.
4. discontinuing all IVs.

(176) 29. The Uniform Anatomical Gift Act:
1. stipulates physicians who certify death shall not be involved in removal or transplant of organs.
2. prohibits selling or purchasing organs.
3. facilitates this area of medical and nursing research.
4. stipulates that at the time of death a qualified health care provider must ask family members to donate organs.

(178) 30. The goal of the Dying Person's Bill of Rights is to:
1. assist the nurses in providing appropriate care.
2. list the treatment options of the patient.
3. provide guidelines for the health care agencies.
4. ensure death with dignity for the patient.

(176) 31. An advance directive:
1. appoints a health care surrogate to make decisions in the event the patient/individual is incompetent.
2. provides for decisions related to the patient's financial needs.
3. describes the patient's wishes about his estate when death is near.
4. describes the patient's wishes about his care when death is near.

(176) 32. The purpose of a living will is to allow people to make decisions regarding their:
1. financial estate.
2. medical care.
3. attending physician.
4. prescription medications.

(176) 33. Durable power of attorney:
1. appoints a health care surrogate to make decisions in the event the patient/individual is incompetent.
2. provides for decisions related to the patient's financial needs.
3. describes the patient's wishes about his estate when death is near.
4. describes the patient's wishes about his care when death is near.

Admission, Transfer, and Discharge

Answer Key: Textbook page references are provided as a guide for answering these questions. A complete answer key was provided for your instructor.

TERMS

Objective

- Define key terms as listed.

Match the terms in Column A with the appropriate definition or description in Column B.

	Column A		Column B
(186)	1. _____ Admission	a.	Systematic process of planning for care after release from a health care facility
(199)	2. _____ Against medical advice	b.	Mental confusion characterized by inadequate or incorrect perception of place, time, and identity
(194)	3. _____ Discharge	c.	Moving a patient from one unit to another
(194)	4. _____ Discharge planning	d.	Fears and apprehension caused by separation from familiar surroundings and significant persons
(186)	5. _____ Disorientation	e.	Entry into healthcare facility
(187)	6. _____ Empathy	f.	Leaving a facility without a physician's order
(186)	7. _____ Health care facility	g.	Leaving a health care facility with a physician's order
(197)	8. _____ Home health agency	h.	Ability to recognize and to some extent share emotions and understand the meaning and significance of another's behavior
(186)	9. _____ Separation anxiety	i.	Any agency that provides health care
(193)	10. _____ Transfer	j.	An organization that provides health care in the home

CLIENT RESPONSE TO HOSPITALIZATION

Objectives

- Describe common patient reactions to hospitalization.
- Identify nursing interventions for common patient reactions to hospitalization.

(186) 11. Provide examples of nursing interventions for the following reactions to hospitalization.

Fear of the unknown _____

Loss of identity _____

Disorientation _____

Separation anxiety/loneliness _____

Multiple Choice

(187) 12. The practical/vocational nurse is aware that separation anxiety can be expressed in older adults by:
1. quietness.
2. crying.
3. calling for the nurse.
4. fear.

(187) 13. The nurse is aware that separation anxiety can be expressed in children by:
1. quietness.
2. crying.
3. calling for the nurse.
4. fear.

(186) 14. Fear of the unknown can be related to Maslow's need for:
1. self-esteem.
2. self-actualization.
3. safety.
4. belonging.

(186) 15. Loss of identity can be related to Maslow's need for:
1. self-esteem.
2. self-actualization.
3. safety.
4. belonging.

ADMISSION

Objective

- Discuss the nurse's responsibilities in performing an admission.

Student Name_____

(187)   16.   Provide the rationale for each of the following nursing actions related to the admission of the patient to the care unit.

         Checking and verifying of ID band. _____

         Assessing immediate needs. _____

         Explaining hospital routines, such as visiting hours, mealtime, and morning

         wake-up. _____

(188)   17.   List the information that should be included when orienting the patient to the room.

TRANSFER

Objective

- Describe how the nurse prepares a patient for transfer to another unit or facility.

(196)   18.   When transferring a patient to another unit or facility the nurse should:

DISCHARGE

Objectives

- Discuss discharge planning.
- Explain how the nurse prepares a patient for discharge.
- Identify the nurse's role when a patient chooses to leave the hospital against medical advice.

(194)   19.   Ideally, discharge planning begins: _____.

(197)   20.   Identify two examples of health care disciplines other than nursing that are involved in referrals and their role in the discharge process.

(199)   21. Provide the rationale for each of the following nursing actions in the discharge of a patient.

Makes certain there is a written discharge order. _____

Arranges for patient and family to visit the business office and check to see that a release

has been given. _____

Notifies the family or person who will be transporting the patient to home.

_____

_____

Gathers equipment, supplies, and prescriptions that the patient is to take home.

_____

_____

Assists the patient in dressing and packing items to go home.

_____

_____

Multiple Choice

(199)   22. When a patient wishes to leave the hospital against medical advice (AMA), the nurse's first responsibility is to:
1. notify the physician.
2. document the incident thoroughly in the nurse's notes.
3. detain the patient.
4. request that the patient sign the special release form (AMA form).

(199)   23. After the patient has been discharged AMA, the nurse:
1. notifies the accounting department.
2. notifies the supervisor.
3. documents the incident thoroughly in the nurse's notes.
4. reports the AMA to the risk manager.

NURSING PROCESS

Objectives

- Identify guidelines for admission, transfer, and discharge of a patient.
- Discuss the nursing process and how it pertains to admitting, discharging, and transferring the patient.

(187)   24. Discuss factors that the nurse should consider when admitting, transferring, or discharging an older adult patient.

Student Name_____

(187)   25.   Identify at least five guidelines that can be used when communicating with patients from various cultural backgrounds during the admission, transfer, or discharge process.

(189)   26.   Match the statements in Column A with the phase of the Nursing Process in Column B.

Column A	**Column B**
Admission	*Nursing Process*

_____   Explanation of procedures

_____   Patient demonstrates decreased anxiety

_____   Admission, collection of subjective and objective data

a.   Assessment
b.   Diagnosis
c.   Planning
d.   Implementation
e.   Evaluation

Transfer

_____   Patient has remained free from injury

_____   Determine level of understanding regarding the purpose of the transfer

_____   Patient will remain stable during transfer

_____   Confirmed the patient's understanding of transfer and procedures through discussion and questions

Discharge

_____   Verified patient's and family's understanding of instruction for discharge

_____   Identified risk factors

_____   Identified needs for health teaching prior to discharge.

CHAPTER 11

Student Name _____

Vital Signs

Answer Key: Textbook page references are provided as a guide for answering these questions. A complete answer key was provided for your instructor.

TERMS

Objective

- Define the key terms as listed.

Match the terms in Column A with the appropriate definition or description in Column B.

	Column A		Column B
(216)	1. _____ Apical pulse	a.	A myocardial contraction that occurs at a regular rhythm but at a rate less than 60 beats per minute.
(213)	2. _____ Bradycardia	b.	The first blood pressure reading—result of left ventricular contractions and the forcing of the blood into the arteries.
(218)	3. _____ Bradypnea		
(219)	4. _____ Diastolic	c.	A myocardial contraction that occurs at a regular rhythm but at a rate greater than 100 beats per minute.
(218)	5. _____ Dyspnea		
(208)	6. _____ Febrile	d.	A measurement of heartbeat taken at the apex, representative of the actual beating of the heart.
(219)	7. _____ Systolic	e.	A respiratory rate less than 12 per minute.
(213)	8. _____ Tachycardia	f.	The second blood pressure reading that is a result of the decreased pressure in the arteries when the ventricles are resting.
		g.	A body temperature that is above normal.
		h.	Difficulty breathing.

PURPOSE AND GUIDELINES

Objectives

- Discuss the importance of accurately assessing vital signs.
- Discuss methods by which the nurse can ensure accurate measurement of vital signs.
- Identify the guidelines for vital sign measurement.
- Discuss frequency of vital signs measurement.
- State the normal limits of each vital sign.
- List the factors that affect vital sign readings.
- Identify the rationale for each step of the vital sign procedures.

(203)   9. Accurate measurement of vital signs provides the nurse with:

10. For the following vital signs, identify factors that may influence them and how they are affected:

(206)   Temperature _____

(213)   Pulse _____

(219)   Respirations _____

(221)   Blood pressure _____

(205)   11. What are the general guidelines for taking vital signs?

TEMPERATURE

Objective

- Accurately assess oral, rectal, axillary, and tympanic temperatures.

(212)   12. The _____ site is considered the *least* accurate site for
temperature measurement.

(205)   13. Identify the sites for temperature measurement and the expected temperature reading for
each.

Student Name_____

(205)   14.   Convert the following temperature readings:

   37° C   =   _____° F

   101.2° F =   _____° C

   39.2° C   =   _____° F

   97.8° F   =   _____° C

(207)   15.   Describe the nursing actions and rationale for temperature measurement.

(211)   16.   What should the nurse do if the patient's temperature is above normal?

Multiple Choice

(205)   17.   A patient's temperature is 93.2° F. This temperature is referred to as:
   1.   febrile.
   2.   hyperthermia.
   3.   hypothermia.
   4.   pyrexia.

(208)   18.   Normal body cells are at risk for damage when the temperature exceeds:
   1.   100.4° F (38° C).
   2.   104.0° F (41° C).
   3.   105.8° F (41° C).
   4.   110.0° F (43.3° C).

(206)   19.   Normal body temperature can change throughout the day. It is important for the nurse to know that the lowest body temperature can occur between the hours of:
   1.   4 PM–6 PM.
   2.   3 PM –6 PM.
   3.   2 AM –9 AM.
   4.   1 AM –4 AM.

(205)   20.   It is important for a nurse to know that normal body temperature can range from:
   1.   96° F–98.2° F (35.6° C–36.8° C).
   2.   98.2° F–99° F (36.8° C–37.2° C).
   3.   97° F–99.6° F (36.1° C–37.5° C).
   4.   96.2° F–100.2° F (35.7° C–37.9° C).

(207)   21. When obtaining a rectal temperature from an adult, the nurse inserts the electronic thermometer probe into the rectum approximately:
1. ½ inch.
2. 1½ inch.
3. 2 inches.
4. 3 inches.

PULSE

Objectives

- List the various sites for pulse measurement.
- Accurately assess an apical pulse, a radial pulse, and a pulse deficit.

(217)   22. Identify the anatomical site for apical pulse measurement.

(215)   23. The radial pulse is found at:

(217)   24. Identify nursing actions to implement if the patient's pulse is not within normal limits.

(215)   25. Describe the nursing actions and rationale for apical and radial pulse measurement.

Multiple Choice

(216)   26. Pulse deficit is described as the difference between the radial and:
1. femoral pulse rate.
2. brachial pulse rate.
3. apical pulse rate.
4. carotid pulse rate.

(214)   27. The patient's pulse is difficult to assess and disappears with slight pressure. The pulse strength is described as:
1. absent.
2. weak.
3. thready.
4. abnormal.

(214)   28. The patient's pulse is easily palpable but disappears when moderate pressure is applied.
The pulse strength is described as:
1. thready.
2. weak.
3. normal.
4. abnormal.

(217)   29. When assessing the apical pulse, the nurse counts pulse rate for:
1. 20 seconds and multiplies by 3.
2. 60 seconds and does not multiply.
3. 30 seconds and multiplies by 2.
4. 15 seconds and multiplies by 4.

RESPIRATION

Objective

- Describe the procedure for determining the respiratory rate.

(220)   30. In determining the respiratory rate, the nurse counts for _____ seconds.

(218)   31. A rapid respiratory rate is described as: _____.

(219)   32. The respiratory rate may be increased by:

(220)   33. Describe the nursing actions and rationale for measurement of respirations.

(219)   34. What should the nurse do if the patient's respirations are rapid and labored?

Multiple Choice

(217)   35. The best definition of internal respiration is the:
1. exchange of gas at the tissue and cell level.
2. exchange of carbon dioxide and oxygen between blood and the lungs.
3. exchange of gas at the alveolar level.
4. cycle of inspiration and expiration.

(218)   36. Respiratory rate is controlled by the:
　　　　　　　1. cerebellum.
　　　　　　　2. spinal cord.
　　　　　　　3. medulla oblongata.
　　　　　　　4. cerebrum.

BLOOD PRESSURE

Objectives

- Accurately assess the blood pressure.
- Describe the benefits of and precautions to follow for self-measurement of blood pressure.

(223)   37. When obtaining the patient's blood pressure, the cuff is deflated at a rate of:

　　　　　　　_____.

(222)   38. The pulsating sounds that are heard when assessing the patient's blood pressure are

　　　　　　　known as _____ sounds.

(222)   39. When should the blood pressure be assessed in the lower extremities?

(223)   40. Describe the nursing actions and rationale for measurement of blood pressure.

(224)   41. What nursing actions should be implemented if the patient's blood pressure is below
　　　　　　　normal?

(225)   42. What are the advantages and disadvantages of self-measurement of blood pressure?

Student Name _____

Multiple Choice

(219)   43.   Hypertension is defined as sustained elevation above:
1.   130/86 mm Hg.
2.   140/70 mm Hg.
3.   140/90 mm Hg.
4.   140/80 mm Hg.

(223)   44.   A high blood pressure reading may result if the blood pressure cuff is:
1.   too large.
2.   too small.
3.   placed low on the arm.
4.   placed high on the arm.

HEIGHT AND WEIGHT

Objective

- Accurately assess the height and weight measurements.

(226)   45.   To obtain an accurate weight measurement, the nurse should:

(227)   46.   Describe the nursing actions and rationale for measurement of height and weight.

(226)   47.   It is important for the nurse to know how to convert a weight in pounds to the equivalent

in kilograms. A patient that weighs 44 lbs is _____ kg.

(226)   48.   Fluid balance may be assessed by weighing the patient. If the patient weighs 1 kg less today
than yesterday, how much fluid was lost?

DOCUMENTATION AND REPORTING

Objectives

- Accurately record and report vital sign measurements.
- State the normal limits of each vital sign.

(227)   49.   Identify the expected vital signs for the following age groups:

	Pulse	**Respirations**	**Blood Pressure**
Neonate			
Toddler			
Adolescent			
Adult			

(227)   50.   In most health care facilities, vital signs are documented on a: _____.

(227)   51.   What vital sign measurements should be reported immediately?

CHAPTER 12 Medical/Surgical Asepsis and Infection Control

Answer Key: Textbook page references are provided as a guide for answering these questions. A complete answer key was provided for your instructor.

TERMS

Objective

- Define the key terms listed.

    1.   Define the following terms:

(236)   Carrier _____

(239)   Endogenous _____

(239)   Exogenous _____

(237)   Fomite _____

(237)   Vector _____

ASEPSIS

Objectives

- Explain the difference between medical and surgical asepsis.
- Identify principles of surgical asepsis.

(232)   2.   Describe the difference between medical and surgical asepsis.

(256)   3.   Identify the seven major principles of sterile technique and provide at least one example for each of how the nurse implements the principle.

INFECTION/INFLAMMATION

Objectives

- Discuss the events in the inflammatory response.
- Describe the signs and symptoms of a localized infection and those of a systemic infection.

(238)   4.   Describe and inflammatory response and the stages of the infectious process.

(238)   5.   Identify the differences between a localized and systemic response to infection.

CHAIN OF INFECTION

Objectives

- Explain how each element of the chain of infection contributes to infection.
- List five major classifications of pathogens.
- Differentiate between *Staphylococcus aureus* and *Staphylococcus epidermidis* regarding virulence.
- Discuss nursing interventions used to interrupt the sequence in the infection process.
- Discuss examples for preventing infection for each element in the chain of infection.

Student Name_____

(232–237)   6.   For the chain of infection, identify how each element contributes to infection and nursing interventions to prevent or control the spread of infection.

	Contribution to Infectious Process	**Nursing Actions**
Infectious agent		
Reservoir		
Exit route		
Method of transmission		
Entrance		
Host		

(234)   7.   Identify the five major classifications of pathogens and one example of a microorganism for each.

(233)   8.   *Staphylococcus aureus* and *Staphylococcus epidermis* differ from in each other in virulence in what way?

(238)   9.   Identify the normal body defense mechanisms and factors that may alter each.

Skin _____

Respiratory tract _____

Gastrointestinal tract _____

Multiple Choice

(236)   10.   The patient has a large midline abdominal incision. To specifically reduce a possible reservoir of infection, the nurse:
1.   wears gloves and mask at all times.
2.   isolates the client's personal articles.
3.   has the client cover the mouth and nose when coughing.
4.   changes the dressing when it becomes soiled.

NOSOCOMIAL INFECTION

Objective

- Explain conditions that promote the onset of nosocomial infections.

(239)   11.   Describe a nosocomial infection and identify conditions that may lead to its development.

INFECTION CONTROL

Objectives

- Demonstrate the appropriate procedure for 2-minute hand washing.
- Discuss the recommended guidelines of isolation precautions for the health care facility, referred to as standard precautions.
- Demonstrate technique for gowning and gloving.
- Demonstrate the procedure for double-bagging contaminated articles.
- Correctly don and remove sterile gloves using the open technique.
- Describe the accepted techniques of preparation for disinfection and sterilization.
- Discuss patient teaching for infection control.

(241)   12.   Identify at least five miscellaneous guidelines for standard precautions.

(242)   13.   Discuss at least four areas for patient teaching to prevent the spread of infection in the home environment.

(242)   14.   You discover that your nursing colleague has an allergy to latex. What should you suggest?

(243)   15.   You are observing the nursing assistant perform hand washing. Identify whether the following actions are appropriate or require more instruction.

Hands are kept higher than the elbows. _____

Faucets are turned off with a dry paper towel. _____

Care is taken to wash around jewelry. _____

(247)   16.   What is the proper method for disposal of sharps?

(247)   17.   For the following patients on isolation precautions, identify the type of room that should be selected:

A client with an active infectious disease _____

A client with an immunosuppressive problem_____

(247)   18.   Identify the basic principles of isolation.

(260)   19.   Identify the proper steps for donning and removing sterile gloves.

(244)   20.   Describe the procedure for gowning for isolation.

(249)   21.   Articles from the patient's isolation room require double-bagging. Identify if the following actions by the nurse are appropriate or inappropriate.

Bag is removed completely from the patient's room. _____

Contaminated bag is dropped into a second bag without touching the edges of the second

bag. _____

Gown, gloves, and mask are removed before double-bagging. _____

(257)   22.   Describe the steps for opening a wrapped sterile package.

(251)   23.   Explain how sterile solutions should be poured onto a sterile field.

(252)   24.   Provide an example of a patient who would require the following precautions:

Airborne precautions _____

Droplet precautions _____

Contact precautions _____

(258)   25.   Discuss how the nurse prepares equipment and surfaces for cleansing, disinfection, and sterilization.

(263)   26.   Identify at least two specific considerations for the older adult client regarding the infectious process.

(264)   27.   Specify two possible nursing diagnoses for a client who is susceptible to or affected by an infectious process.

Student Name_____

Multiple Choice

(252)   28. The nurse is preparing a room for a patient with Herpes simplex virus. The specific aspect for this type of precaution is that the care should include:
1. a private room with negative air flow.
2. hand washing after filtration masks are removed.
3. use of gloves and gown upon entering the room.
4. use of a surgical mask on the patient during transfers.

(252)   29. The nurse is preparing a teaching plan for patients about Rubella. The nurse informs them that this virus may be transmitted by:
1. mosquitoes
2. droplet nuclei.
3. blood products.
4. improperly handled food.

(240)   30. The nurse is working on a unit with a number of patients who have infectious diseases. One of the most important methods for reducing the spread of microorganisms is:
1. sterilization of equipment.
2. the use of gloves and gowns.
3. maintenance of isolation precautions.
4. hand washing before and after client care.

(252)   31. The assignment today for the nurse includes a client with tuberculosis. In caring for a patient on airborne precautions, the nurse should routinely use:
1. regular masks and eyewear.
2. regular masks, gowns, and gloves.
3. surgical hand washing and gloves.
4. filtration masks and gowns.

CHAPTER 13 Safety

Answer Key: Textbook page references are provided as a guide for answering these questions. A complete answer key was provided for your instructor.

TERMS

Objective

- Define the key terms as listed.

    1.   Define or describe the following:

(280)   Disaster situation _____

(271)   Hazard Communication Act _____

(280)   RACE _____

(275)   Safety Reminder Device (SRD) _____

ENVIRONMENT

Objective

- Discuss necessary modifications of the hospital environment for the left-handed patient.

(268)   2.   The patient who has just been admitted to the unit is left-handed. What special instructions will you provide to the nursing assistant for modification of the patient's environment?

PROMOTION OF SAFETY

Objectives

- Relate OSHA's guidelines for violence protection programs to the workplace.
- Summarize safety precautions that can be implemented to prevent falls.

(269)   3.   Identify at least five risk factors for work-related violence in the health care agency and five ways in which the nurse can be involved in violence prevention.

(270)   4.   A patient in the long-term care facility has a history of falls in the home. Identify nursing interventions that may be implemented to prevent falls while the patient resides in the facility.

Multiple Choice

(270)   5.   An older adult patient in the extended care facility has been wandering around outside of the room during the late evening hours. The client has a history of falls. The nurse intervenes by:
1. placing a posey jacket on the patient during the night.
2. keeping the light on and the television playing all night.
3. reassigning the patient to a room close to the nursing station.
4. having the family members come and check on the patient during the night.

(282)   6.   For the nursing diagnosis, *Risk for injury/falls*, identify a patient outcome and three nursing interventions.

Student Name_____

SPECIFIC SAFETY CONCERNS

Objectives

- Relate specific safety considerations to the developmental age and needs of individuals across the life span.
- Identify nursing interventions that are appropriate for individuals across the life span to ensure a safe environment.
- Identify safety concerns specific to the health care environment.

(271)   7.   For the following age groups, identify a specific safety concern and a nursing intervention to prevent injury.

	Safety Concern	Nursing Intervention
Infant		
Toddler		
Older adult		

(270)   8.   Identify basic precautions that may be implemented by the nurse to promote overall safety in the health care environment.

(271)   9.   Describe how the nurse can promote safe ambulation for the patient in a health care facility.

(277)   10. Identify three additional factors that influence the safety of the older adult in the home or health care environment.

(271)   11. What are some of the safety risks to the nurse working within the health care environment?

Multiple Choice

(271)   12. A male patient of average body build resides in the extended care facility and requires assistance to ambulate down the hall. The nurse has noticed that the patient has some weakness to the left side. The nurse assists this patent to ambulate by standing at his:
1.   left side and holding his arm.
2.   right side and holding his arm.
3.   left side and holding one arm around his waist.
4.   right side and holding one arm around his waist.

SAFETY REMINDER DEVICES

Objectives

- Describe safe and appropriate methods for the application of safety reminder devices.
- Discuss nursing interventions that are specific to the patient requiring a safety reminder device.
- Detail measures to create a restraint-free environment.

(272)   13. Identify the related principles for the application and maintenance of safety reminder devices:

Medical orders _____

Patient assessment _____

Maintenance of skin integrity and circulation _____

Documentation _____

Student Name _____

(277)   14. Describe how the nurse may implement a restraint-free environment for a patient.

Multiple Choice

(272)   15. The patient is newly admitted to the extended care facility and appears to be disoriented. There is a concern for the client's immediate safety. The nurse is considering the use of a safety reminder device to prevent an injury. The nurse recognizes that the use of a safety reminder device requires:
1. a physician's order.
2. the patient's consent.
3. a family member's consent.
4. agreement among all of the nursing staff.

FIRE SAFETY

Objective

- Cite the steps to be followed in the event of a fire.

(281)   16. In the event of a fire in a health care agency, the nurse's top priority is: _____.

(281)   17. The nurse is planning to teach a community group about fire safety in the home. What information should be included in the presentation?

(279)   18. There is a fire in the health care agency. Identify the nursing interventions for the following:

A client who is close to the area of the fire but is unable to ambulate _____

Visitors have gone over to use the elevators _____

A client has oxygen in use _____

(279)   19. For the following fires, identify the extinguisher that should be used:

Paper in a wastebasket _____

A liquid anesthetic _____

An electric IV infusion pump _____

Multiple Choice

(279)   20. While walking through the hallway in the hospital, the nurse notices smoke coming from the wastebasket in the patient's room. Upon entering the room, the nurse finds that there is a fire that is starting to flare up. The nurse should first:
   1. extinguish the fire.
   2. remove the patient from the room.
   3. contain the fire by closing the door to the room.
   4. turn off all of the surrounding electrical equipment.

DISASTER PLANNING

Objective

 • Discuss the role of the nurse in disaster planning.

(281)   21. Explain the difference in focus between an internal and external disaster.

(281)   22. What is the role of the nurse in disaster planning?

ACCIDENTAL POISONING

Objective

 • Describe nursing interventions in the event of accidental poisoning.

Student Name_____

(282)   23.   Identify the specific risks for and prevention of accidental poisoning for each group:

	Risks	**Preventive measures**
Children		
Older adults		

(282)   24.   A patient is suspected of having ingested a poisonous substance. The nurse should:

Multiple Choice

(283)   25.   A mother calls the poison control center after a child has ingested a bottle of baby aspirin. The mother should be instructed to:
   1.   identify the amount of substance ingested.
   2.   give the age-appropriate amount of syrup of ipecac.
   3.   position the child, lying down, with the head tilted back.
   4.   drive the child herself to the nearest emergency room.

14 Body Mechanics and Patient Mobility

Student Name _____

Answer Key: Textbook page references are provided as a guide for answering these questions. A complete answer key was provided for your instructor.

TERMS

Objective

- Define the key terms as listed.

Match the terms in Column A with the appropriate definition or description in Column B.

	Column A		Column B
(295)	1. _____ Abduction	a.	Turning the lower arm so that the palm is down
(295)	2. _____ Adduction	b.	Movement of limb away from the body
(298)	3. _____ Contracture	c.	Lying supine with the hips and knees flexed and thighs abducted
(295)	4. _____ Dorsiflexion	d.	Head is positioned lower, with the torso and legs inclined upwards
(295)	5. _____ Flexion	e.	Movement of limb toward axis of the body
(291)	6. _____ Lithotomy	f.	Movement of the joint to decrease the angle between two adjoining bones
(291)	7. _____ Orthopneic	g.	Bend or flex backward
(295)	8. _____ Pronation	h.	Turning the lower arm so that the palm is up.
(295)	9. _____ Supination	i.	Sitting up in bed at a 90-degree angle, perhaps resting forward
(292)	10. _____ Trendelenburg	j.	Abnormal flexion and fixation of a joint

BODY MECHANICS

Objectives

- State the principles of body mechanics.
- Explain the rationale for using appropriate body mechanics.

(288)   11.   Identify four principles of body mechanics for health care workers and the rationale for each one.

(289)   12.   The nurse is observing a colleague performing patient care. Identify if the following techniques are appropriate or inappropriate body mechanics.

Facing away from the work _____

Positioning the feet 6–8 inches apart _____

Keeping the knees straight _____

Keeping the head down _____

Sliding heavy objects _____

Relaxing the abdominal muscles _____

POSITIONING

Objective

- Demonstrate positioning in Fowler's, supine (dorsal), Sims', side-lying, prone, dorsal recumbent, and lithotomy.

(290)   13.   For the following patient positions, identify the position of the bed and the equipment needed and its placement for patient alignment:

	Bed Position	Equipment and Placement for Patient Support
Fowler's		
Supine		
Sims'		

Student Name _____

Bed Position	Equipment and Placement for Patient Support
Side-lying	
Prone	
Dorsal recumbent	
Lithotomy	

(292)   14. What is the rationale for the use of the following devices?

Hand rolls _____

Foot boots _____

Side rails _____

Wedge pillows _____

RANGE OF MOTION

Objective

- Explain range-of-motion exercises.

(295)   15. Identify the purpose and principles related to performance of range-of-motion exercises.

MOVING PATIENTS

Objective

- Relate appropriate body mechanics to the technique for turning, moving, lifting, and carrying the patient.

(298)   16.   Prior to turning or transferring patients, what patient assessment and preparations should be made?

(300)   17.   For the following situations, identify the nursing intervention:

A patient is going to ambulate after not being out of bed for a while.

A patient who is in bed and has a serious head and neck condition needs to be turned.

A patient with left-sided weakness is to move from the bed to a chair.

Multiple Choice

(301)   18.   The nurse is working with a patient who is only able to minimally assist the nurse in moving from the bed to the chair. The nurse needs to help the patient up. The correct technique for lifting the patient to stand and pivot to the chair is to:
1. keep the legs slightly bent.
2. maintain a narrow base with the feet.
3. keep the stomach muscles loose.
4. support the patient away from the body.

(294)   19.   The patient has had a surgical procedure and is getting up to ambulate for the first time. While ambulating down the hallway, the patient complains of severe dizziness. The nurse should first:
1. call for help.
2. lower the patient gently to the floor.
3. lean the patient against the wall until the episode passes.
4. support the patient and move quickly back to the room.

Student Name _____

IMMOBILITY

Objectives

- Discuss the complications of immobility.
- State the nursing interventions to prevent complications of immobility.
- Identify complications caused by inactivity.

(293)   20. Identify the complications of immobility and nursing interventions that may be implemented to prevent their occurrence.

(293)   21. For the following situations, identify the nursing intervention.

The patient develops a reddened area on the sacrum.

While transferring the patient from the bed to a chair, the patient starts to fall.

The client with right-sided weakness following a cerebrovascular accident (CVA or stroke) is unable to perform range of motion of the right extremities.

Multiple Choice

(293)   22. The patient will be immobilized for an extended period of time. The nurse recognizes that there is a need to prevent respiratory complications and intervenes by:
1. suctioning the airway every hour.
2. changing the patient's position every 4–8 hours.
3. using oxygen and nebulizer treatments regularly.
4. encouraging deep breathing and coughing every hour.

(293)   23. Patients who are immobilized in health care facilities require that their psychosocial needs be met along with their physiological needs. The nurse recognizes these needs when telling the patient:
1. "Visiting hours will be limited so you can rest."
2. "We will help you do everything so you don't have to worry."
3. "Let's talk about what you used to do at home during the day."
4. "A private room can be arranged for you."

(292)   24. The patient experienced a CVA that left her with severe left-sided paralysis and very limited mobility. To prevent prolonged dorsiflexion, the nurse uses a:
1. foot boot.
2. bed board.
3. trapeze bar.
4. trochanter roll.

(302)   25. Identify a nursing diagnosis for a patient who has had a CVA with resulting right-sided paresis.

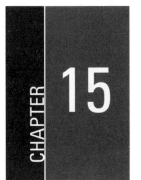

Student Name _____

CHAPTER 15

Pain Control, Comfort, Rest, and Sleep

Answer Key: Textbook page references are provided as a guide for answering these questions. A complete answer key was provided for your instructor.

TERMS

Objective

- Define the key terms listed.

    1. Define or describe the following:

(310)   Endorphin _____

(310)   Gate control theory _____

(309)   Noxious _____

(318)   Patient-controlled analgesia (PCA) _____

(316)   Transcutaneous electrical nerve stimulation (TENS)_____

_____

COMFORT AND DISCOMFORT

Objective

- List 10 possible causes of discomfort.

(308)   2.   Identify at least 10 different causes of discomfort that the nurse should be aware of for the patient in the health care or home environment.

DESCRIPTIONS AND THEORIES OF PAIN

Objectives

- Explain McCaffery's description of pain.
- Explain the relationship of the gate control theory to selecting nursing interventions for pain relief.
- Discuss the synergistic relationship of fatigue, sleep disturbance, and depression to perception of pain.

(309)   3.   McCaffery's description of pain is: _____

_____.

(310)   4.   Using the gate control theory of pain, identify the types of nursing interventions that should be implemented that will be most effective for the patient.

(310)   5.   Identify how the patient's perception of pain is influenced by factors such as fatigue, sleep disturbance, and depression.

ASSESSMENT OF PAIN

Objectives

- Identify subjective and objective data in pain assessment.
- Discuss the concept of making pain assessment the fifth vital sign.
- Explain several scales used to identify intensity of pain.

Student Name_____

(309)   6.   What is the difference between acute and chronic pain?

(313)   7.   Identify at least five objective signs that the patient is experiencing pain.

(313)   8.   What different types of pain intensity scales are used to assess a patient's pain?

What is the benefit of using a scale to assess pain?

(312)   9.   What subjective data may the nurse obtain from the patient regarding his/her pain experience?

(311)   10.   What is the rationale for making pain assessment the fifth vital sign?

(312)   11. Identify examples of cultural and ethnic considerations for pain assessment and management.

(312)   12. The patient has identified to the nurse that she is experiencing pain. What should the nurse do to fully assess the patient's pain?

PAIN THERAPY

Objectives

- Discuss pain mechanisms affected by each analgesic group.
- List six methods for pain control.

(312)   13. Management of pain is required by the _____ (organization).

Identify three of the key concepts included in the standards that are applied to health care facilities.

(315)   14. Identify at least five guidelines for individualizing pain therapy.

(316)   15. Provide two examples of noninvasive pain relief measures.

Student Name_____

(316)   16. For the following drug classifications, identify an example of a specific medication and how the drug affects the pain mechanism:

	Drug Example	**Pain Relief Mechanism**
Nonopioids		
Opioids		
Adjuvant medication		

Multiple Choice

(317)   17. The patent had a surgical procedure this morning and is requesting a pain medication. The nurse assesses the patient's vital signs and decides to withhold the medication based on the finding of:
1. pulse = 90/min.
2. respirations = 8/min.
3. blood pressure = 130/80.
4. temperature = 99° F, rectally.

(316)   18. The visiting nurse is working with a patient who has arthritis. The patient has no known allergies to any medications, so the nurse anticipates that the physician will prescribe:
1. Darvon.
2. Benadryl.
3. ibuprofen.
4. morphine.

NURSING INTERVENTION IN PAIN MANAGEMENT

Objectives

- Discuss the responsibilities of the nurse in pain control.
- Identify nursing interventions to control painful stimuli in the patient's environment.

(312)   19. What problem(s) can occur if the nurse does not respond to and treat the patient's pain?

(319)   20.   What is the role of the nurse in the administration of epidural analgesia?

(315)   21.   Identify nursing interventions that may be implemented to reduce or eliminate the patient's pain.

(318)   22.   There are several patients on the medical unit that are experiencing varying degrees of discomfort. What criteria are used to determine if the patient is a candidate for PCA?

(317)   23.   The nurse wishes to intervene and reduce the discomfort experienced by an older adult patient. What special considerations for pain control need to be made by the nurse for a client in this age group?

Multiple Choice

(319)   24.   The patient is receiving epidural analgesia. The nurse is alert for a complication of this treatment and observes the patient for:
1. diarrhea.
2. hypertension.
3. urinary retention.
4. an increased respiratory rate.

SLEEP AND REST

Objectives

- Describe the differences and similarities between sleep and rest.
- Discuss the sleep cycle, differentiating between NREM and REM sleep.

(320)   25.   Compare and contrast sleep and rest.

(322)   26.   Identify and briefly describe the usual phases and stages of the sleep cycle.

NURSING ASSESSMENT

Objectives

- List six signs and symptoms of sleep deprivation.
- Identify two nursing diagnoses related to sleep problems.

(320)   27.   The nurse suspects that a patient is experiencing sleep deprivation if the nurse observes the following signs and symptoms:

(321)   28.   Identify at least two nursing diagnoses related to sleep problems.

(321)   29.   For each of the following factors, identify how sleep may be affected and why:

	Affect on Sleep	**Reason**
Physical illness		
Anxiety		
Drugs		
Environment		
Nutrition		
Exercise		

NURSING INTERVENTIONS

Objective

•   Outline nursing interventions that promote rest and sleep.

(320)   30.   The patient is experiencing difficulty sleeping while in the hospital. Identify nursing interventions that may be implemented to promote sleep.

Multiple Choice

(320)   31.   The nurse enters the patient's room at 3:00 AM and finds that the patient is awake and sitting up in a chair. The patient tells the nurse that she is not able to sleep. The nurse should first:
1.   obtain an order for a hypnotic.
2.   instruct the patient to return to bed.
3.   provide a glass of warm milk with honey.
4.   ask about ways that have helped her to sleep before.

CHAPTER 16

Complementary and Alternative Therapies

Answer Key: Textbook page references are provided as a guide for answering these questions. A complete answer key was provided for your instructor.

TERMS

Objective

- Define the key terms listed.

      1.   Define or describe the following:

(334)   Imagery _____

(332)   Meridians _____

(332)   Qi _____

TYPES OF THERAPIES

Objectives

- Differentiate between complementary and alternative therapies and allopathic (conventional) medicine.
- Describe how herbs differ from pharmaceuticals.
- Explain how a chiropractic physician treats a patient.
- Describe the principles behind acupuncture and acupressure.
- Explain the difference between acupuncture and acupressure.
- Explain how essential oils may be used to provide aromatherapy.
- Discuss the therapeutic results of yoga.
- Explain the theory of reflexology.
- Describe the possible benefits of magnetic therapy.

(326)   2.   It is estimated that _____% of the population in the United States uses one or more forms of complementary and alternative therapy.

(327)   3.   What are some of the general benefits for the use of complementary and alternative therapies?

(327)   4.   How do herbs differ from pharmaceutical agents?

(328)   5.   Identify at least two commonly taken herbs and their uses.

(331)   6.   The patient asks the nurse what the chiropractic doctor will do for him. Describe the role of the chiropractic physician as you would to the patient.

(332)   7.   What is the different between acupuncture and acupressure? What are the principles underlying these therapies?

(331)   8.   Identify two essential oils used in aromatherapy and their uses.

(334)   9.   What is the principle behind reflexology?

(334)   10.   The patient asks the nurse if "those magnets they sell in the store" are really any good? The nurse responds by telling the patient that magnetic therapy is thought to:

(334)   11.   What are the benefits of the use of imagery?

(336)   12.   The patient is preparing to take a yoga class because she has heard that the positive effects include:

NURSING ASSESSMENT AND INTERVENTIONS

Objectives

- Explain why a thorough health history is important for a patient using complementary and alternative therapies.
- List three conditions when therapeutic massage may be contraindicated.

(326)   13.   The nurse is getting a patient's health history. What should the nurse ask the patient about in regard to complementary and alternative therapies and why is it important to ask?

(330)   14.   The patient is asking about including complementary and/or alternative therapies into the treatment regimen. What information should the nurse include in teaching this patient?

(333)   15.   The nurse is preparing the patient for a therapeutic massage. How should the environment be prepared?

(333)   16.   What assessment findings by the nurse will contraindicate the use of a therapeutic massage?

(334)   17. When is reflexology used with caution or contraindicated for the patient?

(334)   18. Patients with the following health problems should be instructed to avoid the use of magnets:

(335)   19. The nurse is preparing to demonstrate relaxation techniques to the patient. What types of behaviors will the nurse be teaching?

(336)   20. What is the role of the nurse in the use of complementary and alternative therapies?

CHAPTER 17

Hygiene and Care of the Patient's Environment

Answer Key: Textbook page references are provided as a guide for answering these questions. A complete answer key was provided for your instructor.

TERMS

Objective

- Define the key terms listed.

Match the terms in Column A with the appropriate definition or description in Column B.

	Column A		Column B
(345)	1. _____ Canthus	a.	Science of health
		b.	Corner of eye
(359)	2. _____ Cerumen	c.	Ear wax
(351)	3. _____ Erythema	d.	Redness of the skin
		e.	Lightheadedness; fainting
(340)	4. _____ Hygiene		
(344)	5. _____ Syncope		

ENVIRONMENT

Objective

- Discuss the therapeutic hospital room environment.

(341)   6.   What does the nurse need to do to prepare a therapeutic hospital room environment?

HYGIENIC CARE

Objectives

- Describe personal hygienic practices.
- Discuss variations of the bath procedure determined by the patient's condition and physician's orders.
- Perform the procedure for the bed bath successfully.
- Perform the procedures for oral hygiene; shaving; hair care; nail care; and eye, ear, and nose care successfully.
- Perform the procedure for perineal care to the male patient and the female patient successfully.
- Perform the procedure for the back rub successfully.

(343)   7.   Identify the usual daily hygienic care schedule.

(341)   8.   What factors influence a patient's personal hygiene?

(344)   9.   For the following patients, identify how bathing may be affected/altered:

The client is extremely fatigued.

The client is on complete bed rest.

The client has right-sided paralysis following a CVA (stroke).

There is inflammation of the perianal tissue.

Student Name_____

(345)   10.   During a bed bath, identify examples of nursing actions to achieve the following:

         Provision of privacy and patient dignity _____

         Promotion of warmth _____

         Reduction in the spread of microorganisms _____

(350)   11.   In preparing to perform a back rub, the nurse will begin at the patient's:

         _____. The type of strokes to use are: _____.

(355)   12.   Oral hygiene for the unconscious patient includes:

(354)   13.   When is shaving the patient with a straight (blade) razor contraindicated?

(357)   14.   What equipment is needed to provide hair care for the bed-bound patient?

(369)   15.   Describe what information is included in a teaching plan on foot care for a patient newly diagnosed with diabetes mellitus.

(359)   16.   The nurse is evaluating the eye care being provided by a new staff member. Identify whether the following actions are appropriate or inappropriate:

         Removing dried secretions with a dampened cotton ball or gauze. _____

         Using soap and water on a washcloth. _____

         Cleansing the eyes from the outer to the inner canthus. _____

         Washing plastic eyeglass lenses with a special cleaning solution. _____

(359)   17.   The nurse observes the patient performing the following ear care. Identify which behaviors are incorrect and require teaching.

Cleaning the internal auditory canal with a cotton-tipped swab._____

Leaving the hearing aid turned off when not in use. _____

(362)   18.   Describe what should be included in teaching care of the nose.

(360)   19.   When providing perineal care, identify examples of nursing actions to achieve the following:

Promotion of privacy and minimal embarrassment

Facilitating the performance of the procedure

Preventing the spread of microorganisms for the male and female patient

(360)   20.   What patient assessment is completed by the nurse just prior to performing perineal care?

Multiple Choice

(358)   21.   The patient in the hospital requires foot care. The nurse providing foot care should include:
1.   cutting away corns and calluses.
2.   filing toenails straight across
3.   instructing the patient to wear loose shoes.
4.   using alcohol for dryness between the toes.

(356)   22.   The nurse is caring for an older adult patient in the extended care facility. The patient wears dentures and the nurse will delegate their care to the nursing assistant. The nurse instructs the assistant that the patient's dentures should be:
1.   cleaned in hot water.
2.   left in place during the night.
3.   brushed with a soft toothbrush.
4.   wrapped in a soft towel when not worn.

_____

(345)   23. The nurse is working out the patient assignment with the nursing assistant. In delegating the morning care for the client, the nurse expects the assistant to:
1. cut the tangles from the patient's hair.
2. use soap to wash the client's eyes.
3. wash the client's legs with long strokes from the ankle to the knee.
4. place the unconscious client in high Fowler's position to provide oral hygiene.

SKIN ASSESSMENT AND SPECIAL CARE

Objectives

- Discuss the procedures for skin care.
- Identify nursing interventions for the prevention and treatment of decubitus ulcers.

(351)   24. The nurse evaluates that the patient's skin is normal. What observations made by the nurse would contribute to this evaluation?

(351)   25. Identify possible risk factors for development of decubitus (pressure) ulcer.

(353)   26. How can the nurse prevent the development of pressure ulcers?

Identify general guidelines for care of pressure ulcers.

Multiple Choice

(351)   27. The nurse determines, after completing the assessment, that an expected outcome for a patient with impaired skin integrity will be that the skin:
1. remains dry.
2. has increased erythema.
3. tingles in areas of pressure.
4. demonstrates increased diaphoresis.

(353)   28. While completing the bath, the nurse notices a reddened area on the patient's sacrum. The nurse should first:
1. cleanse the skin with alcohol.
2. wash the area with hot water and soap.
3. massage the area vigorously.
4. assess for any other areas of erythema.

BED MAKING

Objectives

- Perform the procedure for making the unoccupied bed successfully.
- Perform the procedure for making the occupied bed successfully.

(362)   29. How can the nurse make the bed as clean and comfortable as possible for the patient?

(366)   30. What are the principles of medical asepsis for bed making?

NURSING INTERVENTION TO ASSIST WITH ELIMINATION

Objective

- Discuss assisting the patient in the use of the bedpan, urinal, and bedside commode.

(362)   31. What equipment is necessary to assist the patient who is not able to use the bathroom facilities?

Student Name _____

(366) 32. How can the nurse assist the patient with elimination?

(366) 33. Identify whether the following characteristics of urine and stool are expected or unexpected:

Pink-tinged urine _____

Urine negative for protein and ketone bodies _____

Clay-colored stool _____

Frequency of stool is three times/day _____

(367) 34. Identify at least two nursing diagnoses related to hygienic care.

CHAPTER 18

Specimen Collection and Diagnostic Examination

Answer Key: Textbook page references are provided as a guide for answering these questions. A complete answer key was provided for your instructor.

TERMS

Objective

- Define the key terms as listed.

Match the terms in Column A with the appropriate definition or description in Column B.

	Column A			Column B
(392)	1.	_____ Culture	a.	A small sample of something
(392)	2.	_____ Expectorate	b.	Left in the bladder after voiding
(385)	3.	_____ Fixative	c.	Secretions from the lungs
(392)	4.	_____ Hemoccult	d.	Inserting a needle into a large vein to obtain a specimen
(391)	5.	_____ Residual urine	e.	Substance used to preserve a specimen
(392)	6.	_____ Sensitivity	f.	A laboratory test involving growing microorganisms in a special medium
(390)	7.	_____ Specimen	g.	A laboratory method to determine the effectiveness of an antibiotic
(392)	8.	_____ Sputum	h.	Blood collection system
(396)	9.	_____ Vacutainer	i.	Test that detects blood in the stool
(396)	10.	_____ Venipuncture	j.	Eject mucous, sputum, or fluids from trachea and lungs

PURPOSE AND GUIDELINES FOR SPECIMEN COLLECTION

Objectives

- Explain the rationales for collection of each specimen listed.
- Discuss guidelines for specimen collection.

(376)   11. Identify the rationale for the collection of each of the specimens identified in the chapter.

(390)   12. Identify the general guidelines for specimen collection and diagnostic examinations.

NURSING ASSESSMENT AND INTERVENTIONS

Objectives

- Identify the role of the nurse when performing a procedure for specimen collection.
- Discuss patient teaching for diagnostic testing.
- State appropriate labeling for a collected specimen.
- Discuss the nursing interventions necessary for proper preparations for a patient having a diagnostic examination.
- List the diagnostic tests for which the nurse should determine whether the patient is allergic to iodine.

(376)   13. What are the general responsibilities of the nurse in specimen collection?

(374)   14. Describe the nursing responsibilities in the general preparation of the patient prior to diagnostic testing.

Student Name_____

(375) 15. Identify at least five areas for patient teaching related to specimen collection and diagnostic testing.

(375) 16. Identify considerations for the older adult in regard to specimen collection and diagnostic testing.

(378) 17. What procedures require that the patient be assessed for an allergy to iodine?

(377) 18. If the patient does develop an allergic reaction to the dye used in a diagnostic test, what signs and symptoms will be observed?

What is the treatment for this allergic reaction?

(378) 19. Identify at least four procedures that require the patient to remain NPO beforehand.

(400) 20. Proper labeling of specimens requires:

(380)   21.   During a bronchoscopy, the most important observation is the patient's:

_____.

Following the bronchoscopy, the patient needs to be assessed for:

_____.

(378)   22.   For the following diagnostic tests, identify at least one preprocedure and one postprocedure nursing intervention that should be implemented.

	Preprocedure	**Postprocedure**
Arteriography		
Barium enema		
Bone scan		
Cardiac catheterization		
Colonoscopy		
Glucose tolerance		
Intravenous pyelogram		
Liver biopsy		
Lumbar puncture		
Magnetic resonance imaging		
Paracentesis		
Ultrasound		

Student Name_____

Multiple Choice

(393) 23. The nurse is using a commercially prepared tube for the collection of an aerobic wound specimen for culture. After collecting the specimen with the swab, the nurse should:
1. place the swab into the collection tube, close it tightly, and keep the specimen warm until it is sent to the laboratory.
2. take the swab and mix it with the special color-changing reagent in the collection tube.
3. place the swab into the collection tube and add the liquid culture medium.
4. crush the ampule at the end of the tube and put the tip of the swab into the solution.

(386) 24. Following a lumbar puncture, the patient tells the nurse that he has a headache. The nurse:
1. reduces the patient's fluid intake.
2. places the patient in low Fowler's position.
3. informs the patient's physician immediately.
4. instructs the patient to lie flat for up to 12 hours.

(389) 25. The patient is to have a thoracentesis performed. The nurse assists the patient to which position for this test?
1. dorsal recumbent
2. supine with the arms held above the head
3. sitting up and leaning over a table
4. side-lying with the knees drawn up

(387) 26. The physician has ordered an MRI for the patient. The patient is concerned about the procedure and requests information from the nurse. The nurse informs the patient to expect:
1. having nothing to eat or drink for 4 hours before the test.
2. hearing humming and loud thumping sounds.
3. minor discomfort to the area being tested.
4. frequent position changes.

GLUCOSE TESTING

Objectives

- List the proper steps for teaching blood glucose self-monitoring.
- List the nursing responsibilities for the glucose tolerance test.

(395) 27. What information is necessary to include in the teaching plan for a newly diagnosed diabetic patient who needs to monitor blood glucose levels?

(384)   28. The patient is scheduled to have a glucose tolerance test. How will you explain this procedure and its preparation to the patient?

What are the nurse's responsibilities during the glucose tolerance test?

Multiple Choice

(395)   29. The nurse is teaching the patient how to collect a specimen for blood glucose monitoring. The patient demonstrates correct technique when:
    1. using the center of the finger for the puncture.
    2. holding the finger upright after puncture.
    3. vigorously squeezing the fingertip after puncture.
    4. touching only the blood to the pad on the test strip.

URINE AND STOOL SPECIMENS

Objectives

- Discuss the procedure for obtaining stool specimens.
- List the proper steps when obtaining urine specimens.

(392)   30. What are the purposes for obtaining stool specimens?

(390)   31. How does urine specimen collection differ depending on the test to be done?

Student Name_____

(394)   32. Identify the basic guidelines for a 24-hour urine collection.

Multiple Choice

(390)   33. Instruction to the patient for collection of a midstream sample includes:
1. use of a clean specimen cup.
2. collection of 200 ml of urine for testing.
3. voiding some urine first and then collecting the sample.
4. washing the perineal area with Betadine before collection.

(393)   34. When obtaining a urine specimen from a patient with an indwelling catheter, the nurse should:
1. apply sterile gloves for the procedure.
2. clamp the drainage tubing for 30 minutes before specimen collection begins.
3. disconnect the catheter from the drainage tubing and collect the urine in a specimen cup.
4. insert a small-gauge needle directly into the catheter tubing to draw up the urine.

ADDITIONAL SPECIMEN COLLECTION

Objectives
- State the correct procedure for collecting a sputum specimen.
- Identify procedure for performing a phlebotomy.
- Identify procedure for performing the electrocardiogram.

(405)   35. The nurse is to perform an ECG (electrocardiogram). Explain the purpose of the test, usual position of the patient, and placement of the electrodes.

(392)   36. To assist the patient to produce a sputum specimen, the nurse instructs the patient the

night before to: _____.

(399)   37. For the collection of a sputum specimen:

Identify the steps of the procedure and rationale for each step.

Specify what type of collection device or equipment is needed.

(397)   38. Prior to performing a venipuncture, the nurse selects and assesses the site to be used. What criteria does the nurse use to determine that the site is acceptable?

(402)   39. How does the nurse apply aseptic technique during a venipuncture?

Multiple Choice

(402)   40. A tourniquet is used when performing a venipuncture. The nurse is aware that the tourniquet should be:
1. tied into a knot.
2. left in place no more than 1–2 minutes.
3. placed 6–8 inches above the selected site.
4. tight enough to occlude the distal pulse.

DOCUMENTATION

Objective

- Document the patient's condition before, during, and after a laboratory or diagnostic test.

(406)   41. After a procedure is completed, what general evaluations of patient status should be done by the nurse?

(376)   42. Give an example of how the nurse should document that a specimen has been obtained or a procedure completed.

Student Name _____

19 Selected Nursing Skills

Answer Key: Textbook page references are provided as a guide for answering these questions. A complete answer key was provided for your instructor.

TERMS

Objective

• Define the key terms as listed.

Match the terms in Column A with the appropriate definition or description in Column B.

	Column A			Column B
(480)	1. _____ Defecation		a.	Presence of air or gas in the intestinal tract
(428)	2. _____ Dehiscence		b.	Open, clear passage
(428)	3. _____ Evisceration		c.	Blood vessel lumen widens
(412)	4. _____ Exudate		d.	Fluid and particles slowly discharged from cells
(480)	5. _____ Flatulence		e.	Elimination of bowel wastes
(444)	6. _____ Induration		f.	Separation of wound edges
(444)	7. _____ Patency		g.	Thin, watery drainage
(414)	8. _____ Sanguineous		h.	Bloody drainage
(414)	9. _____ Serous		i.	Protrusion of abdominal organs through opened incision
(435)	10. _____ Vasodilation		j.	Hardness

ASSESSMENT

Objectives

• Discuss the body's response during each stage of wound healing.
• Identify common complications of wound healing.

(411)   11.   Provide an example for each of the following wound classifications:

Clean _____

Clean-contaminated _____

Contaminated _____

(411)   12.   Describe the following aspects of the stages of wound healing:

	Time Frame	Cellular/Tissue Activity
Inflammatory phase		
Reconstruction phase		
Maturation phase		

(412)   13.   Describe the following types of wound healing:

Primary intention _____

Secondary intention _____

Tertiary intention _____

(413)   14.   Identify factors that may impair wound healing.

(419)   15.   Describe the complications that may occur with wound healing and the nursing assessment and intervention for each.

WOUND CARE, SUPPORT, AND COMFORT MEASURES

Objectives

- Explain the procedure for applying sterile dry dressing and wet-to-dry dressings.
- Identify the procedure for removing sutures and staples.
- Discuss care of the patient with a wound drainage system such as Hemovac/Davol suction or T-tube drainage.
- Identify the procedure for performing sterile wound irrigation.
- Discuss the application of bandages and binders.
- Discuss heat and cold therapy/procedures.

Student Name _____

(414)   16.   What is the purpose of each of the following types of dressings?

Gauze _____

Semiocclusive _____

Occlusive _____

(415)   17.   For the following dressings, identify the type of wound that it can be used on:

Dry dressing _____

Wet-to-dry _____

Transparent _____

(416)   18.   You are observing a new staff member perform a sterile dry dressing change. What actions require correction?

The tape is loosened in a direction away from the incision. _____

Clean gloves are used to remove the old dressing. _____

The area surrounding the incision is cleansed, then the incision is cleansed using a back-and-forth stroking motion. _____

Montgomery straps are used. _____

(418)   19.   The new staff member proceeds to do a wet-to-dry dressing change. What actions require correction?

The old dressing is moistened for easy removal. _____

The new dressing is left dripping wet. _____

The deep wound is packed using forceps. _____

A dry dressing is applied over the wet gauze. _____

(419)   20.   The nurse is preparing to implement wound irrigations.

The purpose of wound irrigation is: _____.

The equipment needed for irrigation includes: _____.

The position of a syringe for irrigation is: _____.

The direction of cleansing is: _____.

A hand-held shower is positioned: _____.

(423)   21. The nurse is assessing the amount of drainage that the patient has from a surgical wound and finds that 650 cc has drained from 9:00 AM until now, 11:40 PM. What should the nurse do?

(422)   22. Discuss the specific interventions for irrigating a deep wound.

(424)   23. For staple or suture removal:

Sterile or clean procedure? _____

All of the staples are removed at once? _____

Steri-strips are applied to the site? _____

Intermittent sutures are snipped at skin level away from the knots? _____

(425)   24. Identify two nursing diagnoses associated with wound healing.

(426)   25. What is the difference between a Penrose drain and a Hemovac or Jackson-Pratt drainage system?

(429)   26. What nursing assessment and patient teaching are necessary for a patient with a wound drainage system?

(434)   27. Identify at least three home care considerations for wound care.

(426)   28. Prior to a bandage or binder being applied, what should the nurse assess?

Student Name _____

(434) 29. Identify at least five guidelines for bandage and binder application.

(433) 30. Identify the type of bandage turns that should be used for the following body areas:

Finger or wrist _____

Calf or thigh _____

Joints _____

Scalp _____

(430) 31. The patient is to have an abdominal binder applied. What is an important consideration for the nurse when implementing this application?

(435) 32. Provide examples of the types of hot and cold applications that may be used.

(435) 33. When is the use of hot or cold therapy contraindicated for a patient?

(439) 34. Identify at least four safety measures to be considered when applying hot or cold therapy.

(440) 35. Prior to the application of a hot moist compress to an open wound, the nurse may

apply_____ around the wound to protect the skin.

(442) 36. What materials can the patient use in the home to make a quick ice pack?

Multiple Choice

(435)   37.   A cold application is ordered for the patient. The nurse is aware that a positive effect of this treatment is:
1.   vasodilation.
2.   local anesthesia.
3.   reduced blood viscosity.
4.   increased capillary permeability.

(440)   38.   There are principles to consider when using hot and cold therapy for patients. The nurse recognizes that the:
1.   application usually lasts only 10–20 minutes.
2.   patient should be able to adjust the temperature settings.
3.   patient should be able to move the application around.
4.   application is positioned so that the patient cannot move away from the temperature source.

(426)   39.   A binder is used for a patient to:
1.   reduce ventilatory capacity.
2.   assist in ambulation.
3.   increase circulatory stasis.
4.   provide support.

(421)   40.   The nurse is preparing to remove the patient's staples. Upon assessment, the nurse determines that the staples should not be removed because:
1.   the wound edges are separated.
2.   there is no drainage from the incision.
3.   the client is anxious about their removal.
4.   a negative cosmetic result could occur.

(415)   41.   The nurse is preparing to change the patient's dry sterile dressing. Upon attempting the removal of the old dressing, it is found to be adhered to the site. The nurse should:
1.   notify the physician.
2.   leave the dressing in place.
3.   pull the dressing off quickly.
4.   moisten the dressing with saline.

IRRIGATIONS

Objectives

- Identify the procedure for irrigating the eye and the ear.
- Explain the procedure for external and internal vaginal irrigation (douche).
- Discuss the procedure for nasal irrigation.

Student Name_____

(436)   42.   For an eye and ear irrigation, identify the following:

	Eye irrigation	**Ear irrigation**
Position of patient		
Position of irrigating equipment		
Flow of solution		
Postprocedure care		

(475)   43.   The nurse is preparing to perform a vaginal irrigation for a patient.

Perineal care is required before the irrigation if the patient has:

_____.

The patient is positioned in bed on a: _____.

The temperature of the irrigating solution is: _____.

Medical or surgical asepsis is used? _____

While inserting the irrigating nozzle, the nurse should:

_____.

(491)   44.   A nasal irrigation is being performed on a patient by a nursing colleague. Which steps are appropriate?

Positioning the patient with the head back. _____

Informing the patient not to speak or swallow during the procedure. _____

Inserting the tip of the irrigating device ½–1 inch. _____

Having the patient blow the nose immediately after the irrigation. _____

PARENTERAL THERAPY

Objectives

- Summarize the nurse's responsibilities for the patient receiving intravenous therapy/procedures.
- Explain the nurse's responsibility when administering blood therapy.

(442)   45.   Identify three guidelines for monitoring IV (intravenous) therapy.

(443)   46.   Prior to a venipuncture, what does the nurse need to assess?

(444)   47.   What documentation is necessary following an IV insertion?

(444)   48.   The patient has an IV infusion. What assessments at the insertion site would indicate that the infusion should be discontinued?

(448)   49.   For the following situations, what should the nurse do?

There is less than 100 ml left in the IV bag.

Blood components will be given IV to the patient.

You are unsuccessful on the venipuncture attempt.

The patient asks if the IV insertion will hurt.

(449)   50.   What are the priority nursing responsibilities for a blood transfusion?

(450)   51.   The nurse determines that the patient is having a transfusion reaction. What signs and symptoms did the patient most likely exhibit to lead the nurse to this determination?

What should the nurse do for the patient with a reaction?

Student Name _____

Multiple Choice

(444)   52.   Just prior to IV insertion, the nurse should:
1.   shave the hair from the selected site.
2.   select a proximal site on the upper extremity.
3.   apply a tourniquet 4–6 inches above the site to be used.
4.   vigorously massage the extremity to be used.

(448)   53.   Upon assessment of the IV insertion site, the nurse suspects that the patient has phlebitis. This is based upon the observation of:
1.   edema at the site.
2.   erythema along the vein path.
3.   cool skin around the insertion site.
4.   an increase in systemic blood pressure and pulse.

(449)   54.   A blood transfusion is prepared for the patient. In setting up the IV, the nurse is aware that an acceptable piggyback solution for the set is:
1.   normal saline.
2.   5% dextrose in water.
3.   10% dextrose in water.
4.   Ringer's solution.

OXYGENATION

Objectives

- Discuss nursing interventions/procedures for the patient receiving oxygen.
- Discuss care of (procedures for) a patient with a tracheostomy.
- Differentiate among oropharyngeal, nasopharyngeal, and nasotracheal suctioning.

(451)   55.   Identify at least four safety precautions for oxygen use in the hospital and home environment.

(452)   56.   The patient is to receive oxygen. What assessments should be made by the nurse?

(457)   57.   When performing tracheostomy care, the nurse is aware of the following:

Cleansing solution to be used _____

Rinsing solution to be used _____

The part that is removed for cleaning _____

Safety measures _____

(456)   58.   What can the nurse do to reduce possible sensory deprivation for the patient with a tracheostomy?

(456)   59.   What criteria are used for the reinflation of a tracheostomy cuff?

(462)   60.   In preparing to suction a patient, the nurse implements the following:

Position of patient, if able _____

Appropriate vacuum pressure for adult patient _____

Check the patency of suction catheter tubing by _____

Lubricant used on tubing _____

Length of insertion for nasotracheal suctioning for adult patient _____

Suctioning performed for _____ seconds

Multiple Choice

(457)   61.   The patient requires suctioning of pulmonary secretions. An appropriate nursing diagnosis for this patient is:
1.   Fluid volume excess.
2.   Ineffective breathing patterns.
3.   Diminished respiratory ability.
4.   Ineffective airway clearance.

(462)   62.   The nurse is working in the special care nursery and will be suctioning the airways of infants. For this age group, the pressure of the wall suction should be set at:
1.   5–15 mm Hg.
2.   20–40 mm Hg.
3.   50–95 mm Hg.
4.   100–120 mm Hg.

(457)   63.   Preparation for tracheostomy care in the acute care environment includes:
1.   using clean technique and supplies for cleaning.
2.   placing the patient in supine position.
3.   removing and cleaning the outer cannula.
4.   preparing cotton swabs with hydrogen peroxide and saline.

_____

URINARY ELIMINATION

Objective

- Discuss management of the patient with an indwelling catheter:

  Male catheterization
  Female catheterization
  Discontinuing an indwelling catheter
  Catheter irrigation
  Urostomy care

(464)   64.   Identify at least five nursing interventions for patients with urinary drainage systems.

(465)   65.   For urinary catheterization of a male and female patient, identify the following:

	Male	**Female**
Position of patient		
Method of cleansing before insertion		
Length of catheter insertion		

(465)   66.   The nurse is inserting a urinary catheter and encounters the following situations. What should be done?

Resistance is met _____

The male patient has an erection _____

The catheter is inserted into the vagina _____

(465)   67.   The catheter itself is checked before insertion by: _____.

(468)   68.   After catheter removal, the nurse assesses the patient for:

(469)   69.   Describe catheter care for a male and female patient.

(470)   70.   The patient who self-catheterizes at home uses _____ technique.

(470)   71.   What are the different methods of bladder irrigation?

(471)   72.   The patient is receiving continuous bladder irrigation through a three-way indwelling urinary catheter. Ordered: 350 ml of normal saline irrigating solution infused. There are 475 ml in the urinary drainage bag. What is the patient's urinary output?

(484)   73.   The primary concern for a patient with a urostomy is:

(474)   74.   Identify two nursing diagnoses for a patient with a urinary disorder.

Multiple Choice

(467)   75.   The nurse has inserted the catheter into the patient and while inflating the balloon the patient expresses discomfort. The nurse should:
1.   remove the catheter and begin the procedure again.
2.   pull back on the catheter to determine tension.
3.   draw fluid back out from the balloon and move the catheter forward.
4.   continue to inflate the balloon as discomfort is expected.

(469)   76.   The nurse is providing instruction to the nursing assistant on catheter care for the patient. An appropriate instruction is to:
1.   maintain strong tension on the external catheter tubing.
2.   empty the drainage bag every 24 hours.
3.   keep the drainage bag on the bed or attached to the side rails.
4.   clean from the urinary meatus down the catheter.

(467)   77.   When inserting a urinary catheter into a female patient, the nurse knows that it should be inserted:
1.   2–4 inches.
2.   4–6 inches.
3.   6–8 inches.
4.   8–10 inches.

BOWEL ELIMINATION

Objective

- Identify the procedures for promoting bowel elimination:

    Administering an enema
    Inserting a rectal tube
    Performing ostomy/stoma care
    Removing a fecal impaction

Student Name_____

(480)   78.   How can the nurse promote normal bowel functioning for the patient in a hospital or extended care facility?

(485)   79.   The nurse is observing the patient at home performing colostomy care. What areas require further teaching?

The patient says he is not concerned about the swelling of the stoma. _____

Alcohol and skin cream are used around the stoma. _____

The patient is blotting the skin dry around the stoma. _____

The skin barrier and pouch are being changed twice daily. _____

The patient is leaving $\frac{1}{16}$" clearance between the stoma and skin barrier. _____

750 ml of warm water is prepared for the irrigation. _____

The irrigation cone is pushed forcefully into the stoma to create the fit. _____

(486)   80.   For the administration of an enema, the nurse is aware of the following:

Preferred position of patient _____

Temperature of prepared solution _____

Maximum volume of solution for an adult patient _____

Client instruction for relaxation of external sphincter_____

Height of fluid container _____

Length of insertion of tube for adult patient _____

Client complains of cramping _____

Documentation required _____

Multiple Choice

(488)   81.   Prior to the digital removal of a fecal impaction, the nurse checks the medical record. Because of the possible effect of the digital manipulation, a patient with a history of which of the following will have to be observed especially closely during the procedure?
1.   cardiac disease
2.   abdominal discomfort
3.   urinary infection
4.   diabetes mellitus

ENTERAL THERAPY

Objectives

- Explain nursing interventions for the patient with nasogastric intubation.
- Discuss gastric and intestinal suctioning care.
- Identify the procedure for nasogastric tube removal.

(477)   82. What is the purpose of nasogastric (N/G) tube insertion?

(478)   83. The nurse is preparing to perform a N/G tube insertion and is aware of the following:

Measurement for insertion _____

Position of patient for insertion _____

Instructions for patient during insertion _____

Most reliable determination of tube placement _____

Securing of N/G tube _____

(479)   84. The patient is not able to talk after the N/G tube is inserted. The nurse suspects:

(481)   85. You are evaluating the new staff member's performance of a N/G tube irrigation. Which actions indicate that further instruction is needed?

The nurse draws up 100 ml of tap water for the irrigation. _____

The solution is instilled slowly. _____

The solution is withdrawn and measured. _____

Solution is forced down afterward to clear the tubing. _____

(480)   86. The patient is to have gastric or intestinal suctioning applied. Identify the appropriate nursing interventions.

Pressure to set the wall suction at: _____.

Assessment of the patient:

Patency of the Salem sump determined by:

Abnormalities reported to the physician:

(483)   87. While removing the N/G tube, the patient begins to gag. The nurse should:

Student Name _____

Basic Nutrition and Nutritional Therapy

Answer Key: Textbook page references are provided as a guide for answering these questions. A complete answer key was provided for your instructor.

TERMS

Objective

- Define the key terms listed.

1. Define the following terms:

(503)   Anabolism _____

(518)   Basal metabolic rate (BMR) _____

(502)   Catabolism _____

(499)   Essential nutrients _____

(502)   Nitrogen balance _____

(502)   Vegan _____

ESSENTIAL NUTRIENTS

Objectives

- List the six classes of essential nutrients and identify those that provide energy.
- List the functions and food sources of protein, carbohydrates, and fats.
- List food sources and possible health benefits of dietary fiber.
- Distinguish between saturated and unsaturated fats and cholesterol; identify current recommendations for dietary intake of fats and cholesterol.
- Discuss key vitamins and minerals, their role in health, and their food sources.

(499)   2.   Identify the six classes of nutrients and their general function.

(499)   3.   What are the calories provided and the recommended percentage of intake for each of the following nutrients?

Protein _____

Carbohydrates _____

Fats _____

(499)   4.   Identify the following for carbohydrates:

Role in the body _____

Types _____

(500)   5.   Identify an example of a simple and a complex carbohydrate.

(500)   6.   What is the difference between these types of fiber?

Insoluble fiber _____

Water-soluble fiber _____

(500)   7.   What do fats provide for the body?

Student Name _____

(501)　　8.　Identify examples of food sources for the following:

　　　　　　　Saturated fats _____

　　　　　　　Unsaturated fats _____

(501)　　9.　In considering food choices, the nurse recognizes that cholesterol is found mainly in:

　　　　　　_____.

(501)　　10.　Lipoproteins have been talked about in the news. Which ones are important in cardiovascular disease?

(502)　　11.　What is the role of protein in the body?

(502)　　12.　Define and identify possible food sources for a complete protein.

(503)　　13.　For the following types of protein-kilocalorie malnutrition states, describe the problem and the signs and symptoms exhibited by the patient.

　　　　　　　Kwashiorkor _____

　　　　　　　Marasmus _____

(503)　　14.　What is the general function of vitamins?

(503)　　15.　What are the two main types of vitamins?

(503)　　16.　How do minerals differ from vitamins?

(504) 17. For each of the following vitamins, identify a food source, its function in the body, and signs and symptoms of a deficiency and toxicity (if applicable).

Vitamin C

Vitamin D

Vitamin K

Folic Acid

Niacin

(504) 18. The patient tells the nurse that he has heard about antioxidants but is not sure what they are. The nurse responds by telling the patient that antioxidants are:

(511) 19. For a patient over the age of 50, vitamin _____ is recommended.

(506) 20. For each of the following minerals, identify a food source, its function in the body, and signs and symptoms of a deficiency and toxicity (if applicable):

Calcium

Potassium

Iron

Iodine

Zinc

Student Name_____

(509)   21. Identify factors that enhance the absorption of iron.

(510)   22. What is the function of water in the body and the recommended daily intake?

Multiple Choice

(511)   23. The vitamin to be avoided or used with caution for a patient who is taking anticoagulants is vitamin:
         1. A.
         2. D.
         3. K.
         4. B complex.

(504)   24. Patients who have an inadequate intake of vitamin C may develop:
         1. bleeding gums.
         2. liver damage.
         3. depression.
         4. convulsions.

(505)   25. The patient has been diagnosed with pernicious anemia. The nurse expects that the patient will receive:
         1. vitamin B_1.
         2. vitamin B_6.
         3. vitamin B_{12}.
         4. niacin.

(502)   26. The nurse is working with a patient who requires an increase in complete proteins in the diet. The nurse will recommend the intake of:
         1. cereal.
         2. beans.
         3. milk.
         4. vegetables.

(505)   27. A patient in the clinic is asking the nurse about vitamin supplements. The nurse cautions the patient about potential toxicity and not to exceed the guidelines for:
         1. vitamin A.
         2. vitamin B.
         3. vitamin C.
         4. folic acid.

(507) 28. The patient tells the nurse that the ads on television are talking about zinc and its importance. The patient says that he doesn't know anything about zinc and would like to find out what foods have it. The nurse tells the patient that a good source of zinc is:
1. fruit.
2. liver.
3. poultry.
4. cheese.

DIET MODIFICATIONS

Objectives

- Identify standard hospital diets and modifications for texture, consistency, and meal frequency.
- List medical/surgical conditions that require a high-kilocalorie and high-protein diet, and suggest ways to increase kilocalories and protein in the diet.
- Define obesity. List components of an effective weight management program.
- Describe the diet in the treatment of type 1 and type 2 diabetes mellitus.
- Distinguish among anorexia nervosa, bulimia nervosa, and binge eating disorder.
- List conditions requiring a fat-modified diet, and identify foods and food preparation methods that should be limited.
- Identify medical/surgical conditions requiring modifications in sodium, potassium, protein, or fluid intake, and describe the dietary adjustments necessary in these conditions.

(517) 29. Identify what health problems the following diets are used for:

Soft/low residue _____

High kilocalorie _____

(519) 30. What is the body mass index (BMI) used for?

(519) 31. Identify the risks associated with obesity.

(520) 32. What is the general dietary approach for the obese patient?

Student Name_____

(521)   33. Identify the similarities among the eating disorders.

(523)   34. What physiological signs and symptoms should the nurse be alert for that may indicate an eating disorder?

(524)   35. What are the general dietary guidelines for a patient with type 2 diabetes mellitus?

(525)   36. The patient with diabetes mellitus is diaphoretic, weak, and breathing shallowly. What should the nurse do?

(525)   37. What is the 15/15 rule for diabetic patients?

(525)   38.   Describe dumping syndrome and ways that the patient may avoid it.

(526)   39.   Low-fat diets are used for patients with: _____.

(528)   40.   How is the patient able to modify the intake of the following fats?

Eggs _____

Meats _____

(525)   41.   A protein-restricted diet is used for patients with:

_____.

(529)   42.   A sodium-restricted diet is used for patients with:

_____.

(530)   43.   Identify the dietary modifications for patients with the following health problems:

AIDS _____

Constipation _____

Hiatal hernia _____

Multiple Choice

(517)   44.   A patient in the hospital who is placed on a clear liquid diet may have:
1.   fruit juice.
2.   gelatin.
3.   sherbet.
4.   strained soup.

(524)   45.   The nurse recognizes that the diet for a patient diagnosed with diabetes mellitus will be:
1.   fat-modified.
2.   sodium-restricted.
3.   protein-restricted.
4.   carbohydrate-modified.

(536)   46.   A patient who is lactose intolerant needs to avoid:
1.   meat.
2.   fish.
3.   cheese.
4.   vegetables.

ENTERAL THERAPY

Objective

- Define enteral nutrition and parenteral nutrition and list medical/surgical conditions in which nutrition support may be indicated.

(531)   47. What are the indications for the use of enteral feeding?

(531)   48. What are the possible complications of enteral feeding?

(532)   49. What is parenteral nutrition and when is it used?

(537)   50. Complications of parenteral nutrition include:

(533)   51. Identify the nursing assessments and interventions for enteral feeding:

Patient assessment prior to feeding _____

Assessment of gastric aspirate _____

Gastric residual above 150 ml_____

Formula is cold _____

Occlusion of the tubing is suspected _____

After feeding is given _____

Documentation _____

(537)   52. What is included in the care of a gastrostomy or jejunostomy site?

(537)   53. Positive outcomes for patients with enteral tube feedings are:

Multiple Choice

(536)   54. Patients with nasogastric tubes may develop otitis media. In order to prevent this occurrence, the nurse will:
1. increase fluid intake.
2. remove and reinsert the tube q24h.
3. suction the nose and mouth.
4. turn the patient side to side q2h.

(536)   55. A patient on the unit has a N/G tube in place with continuous feedings. When the nurse enters the room, the patient says that he is having stomach cramps. The nurse should first:
1. cool the formula.
2. remove the N/G tube.
3. use a different type of formula.
4. decrease the administration rate.

NURSING ASSESSMENT AND INTERVENTIONS

Objectives

- Discuss the role of the nurse in promoting good nutrition.
- Explain how to use diet planning guides in the assessment and planning of a diet.
- Discuss changes in nutrient needs throughout the life cycle and suggest ideas to ensure adequate nutrition during each stage of life.
- Identify the effects of common medications on nutritional status.

(497)   56. Identify the role of the nurse in promoting nutrition.

(497)   57. In the food pyramid guide, the emphasis is on: _____.

(497)   58. Identify the number of daily servings recommended in the food pyramid for:

Vegetables _____

Meat, poultry, fish _____

Dairy products _____

Student Name _____

(498)   59.   A teenage girl asks the nurse how many calories she should have every day and what types of food she should eat. The nurse provides the following information:

Calorie intake _____

Servings of bread _____

Servings of vegetables _____

Servings of fruit _____

Servings of milk _____

Servings of meat _____

(498)   60.   The main dietary guidelines for Americans are:

(502)   61.   A patient is asking about a vegetarian diet. Explain what the positive and negative aspects of this diet for the patient.

(511)   62.   There is an increased need for nutrients during pregnancy because:

(511)   63.   What vitamins are recommended to be increased for the pregnant patient?

(512)   64. The nurse teaches the pregnant woman to avoid the following foods and lifestyle activities:

(513)   65. In teaching a new parent about nutritional guidelines for the infant, the nurse explains that the following foods should be avoided during the first year:

(514)   66. Identify ways to encourage good dietary habits in children.

(514)   67. A common nutritional problem in adolescence is that a large part of the diet may be comprised of:

(514)   68. Nursing home residents may have nutritional problems as a result of:

(539)   69. You are evaluating the nursing assistant feeding a patient. Identify which of the following actions require correction:

Offering the patient the bedpan before the meal. _____

Placing the patient in low Fowler's position. _____

Using a straw for liquids. _____

Directing food toward the patient's paralyzed side. _____

Talking with the patient during the feeding. _____

Student Name _____

Multiple Choice

(513)   70. The mother asks the nurse about giving strained fruits to her infant. The nurse tells the mother that this food should be introduced at around:
1. 2 months.
2. 5 months.
3. 8 months.
4. 12 months.

(516)   71. The patient is taking a diuretic medication every day. The nurse observes the patient for signs of a decrease in:
1. vitamin K.
2. vitamin C.
3. phosphorus.
4. potassium.

Student Name _____

Fluids and Electrolytes

Answer Key: Textbook page references are provided as a guide for answering these questions. A complete answer key was provided for your instructor.

TERMS

Objective

- Define the key terms listed.

Match the terms in Column A with the appropriate definition or description in Column B.

	Column A		Column B
(548)	1. _____ Active transport	a.	Movement of particles through a solution or gas
(548)	2. _____ Anion	b.	Transfer of water and dissolved substances from an area of higher pressure to an area of lower pressure
(548)	3. _____ Cation		
(547)	4. _____ Diffusion	c.	Solution of higher osmotic pressure
		d.	Force that moves molecules into cells using energy
(548)	5. _____ Electrolyte	e.	Minerals or salts in solution having electrical charges
(548)	6. _____ Filtration	f.	Negatively charged ion
(547)	7. _____ Hypertonic	g.	Solution of the same osmotic pressure
		h.	Positively charged ion
(547)	8. _____ Hypotonic	i.	Solution of lower osmotic pressure
(547)	9. _____ Isotonic	j.	Movement of water from an area of lower concentration to an area of higher concentration
(547)	10. _____ Osmosis		

FLUID AND PARTICLE MOVEMENT

Objectives

- List, describe, and compare the body fluid compartments.
- Discuss active and passive transport processes and give two examples of each.

(545)   11. Most of the body fluid in an adult is located in the _____ compartment.

(546)   12. What is the relationship of body weight to fluid?

(547)   13. For the following types of fluids, identify the how the fluid will move:

Hypertonic solution _____

Hypotonic solution _____

(548)   14. Provide examples for each of the following processes in the body:

Diffusion _____

Filtration _____

Osmosis _____

Active transport _____

ELECTROLYTES

Objectives

- Discuss the role of specific electrolytes in maintaining homeostasis.
- Describe the cause and effect of deficits and excesses of sodium, potassium, chloride, calcium, magnesium, phosphorus, and bicarbonate.

(549)   15. The major extracellular electrolyte is: _____.

The major intracellular electrolyte is: _____.

(549)   16. Identify the most common signs and symptoms of hyponatremia and nursing interventions for the imbalance.

Student Name_____

(551)　　17. Identify the most common signs and symptoms of hypokalemia and nursing interventions for the imbalance.

(552)　　18. What are the most serious problems associated with hyperkalemia and the nursing interventions for the imbalance?

(552)　　19. The role of calcium in the body is:

(553)　　20. Identify the most common signs and symptoms of hypocalcemia and the nursing interventions for the imbalance.

　　　　　　　What special assessments should the nurse perform to determine the presence of this imbalance?

(555)　　21. Identify possible causes of hypomagnesemia, common signs and symptoms, and nursing interventions for the imbalance.

(549)   22. For the following lab results, identify the electrolyte imbalance:

   Serum sodium—127 mEq/L: _____

   Serum potassium—5.6 mEq/L: _____

   Serum calcium—3.8 mEq/L: _____

   Serum magnesium—2.7 mEq/L: _____

Multiple Choice

(552)   23. The patient is experiencing hyperkalemia. The nurse anticipates that the treatment will include:
   1.   IV calcium.
   2.   fluid restrictions.
   3.   foods high in potassium.
   4.   administration of diuretics.

(553)   24. Following an auto accident and a significant hemorrhage, the patient was given a large infusion of citrated blood. The patient is assessed for the development of:
   1.   urinary retention.
   2.   poor skin turgor.
   3.   increased blood pressure.
   4.   positive Chvostek's sign.

ACID-BASE

Objectives

- Differentiate between the roles of the buffers, lungs, and kidneys in maintenance of acid-base balance.
- Describe the four major types of acid-base imbalances.

(556)   25. The pH range of the blood is: _____.

(556)   26. In determining acid-base balance, the base substance that increases or decreases in the

   blood is: _____.

   The acid substance is: _____.

   The ratio of these two substances is: _____.

(556)   27. What are the three body systems that regulate acid-base balance in the body?

Student Name _____

(557) 28. If carbonic acid increases in the blood, the pH will: _____.

The respiratory system will respond by: _____.

(557) 29. If the pH of the blood increases, the kidneys will respond by

_____.

Multiple Choice

(559) 30. The patient has experienced a prolonged episode of diarrhea. The nurse is observing the patient for signs of:
1. metabolic acidosis.
2. metabolic alkalosis.
3. respiratory acidosis.
4. respiratory alkalosis.

(558) 31. The patient has had emphysema for a number of years. Which of the following arterial blood gas values indicates that the patient is in respiratory acidosis?
1. pH 7.35, $PaCO_2$ 40, HCO_3 22
2. pH 7.40, $PaCO_2$ 45, HCO_3 30
3. pH 7.30, $PaCO_2$ 50, HCO_3 24
4. pH 7.48, $PaCO_2$ 55, HCO_3 18

(557) 32. While in the delivery room with his wife, the father-to-be begins to develop an anxiety reaction and lightheadedness. Nursing intervention to prevent respiratory alkalosis is:
1. lay him down.
2. provide nasal oxygen.
3. have him breathe into a paper bag.
4. have him cough and deep-breathe.

(559) 33. A child has gotten into the medicine cabinet in the home and ingested the remaining contents of an aspirin bottle. The problem that may occur as a result of this ingestion is:
1. metabolic acidosis.
2. metabolic alkalosis.
3. respiratory acidosis.
4. respiratory alkalosis

NURSING

Objectives

- Discuss the role of the nursing process for fluid, electrolyte, and acid-base balances.
- Discuss how the very young, the very old, and the obese patient are at risk for fluid volume deficit.

(545)   34.   How does body fluid change as an individual ages and grows?

(545)   35.   Identify at least two considerations for the older adult patient regarding fluid and electrolyte and acid-base balance.

(547)   36.   The nurse is monitoring the patient's intake and output (I & O). What should be counted as part of the output?

(558)   37.   What are the signs and symptoms of respiratory acidosis?

(557)   38.   The nurse anticipates that the treatment for respiratory acidosis will include:

Student Name _____

(559) 39. Identify possible causes of and interventions for metabolic acidosis and alkalosis.

(559) 40. Identify possible nursing diagnoses and outcomes for patients experiencing fluid, electrolyte, or acid-base imbalances.

(560) 41. What are the nursing interventions that should be implemented for patients with fluid, electrolyte, or acid-base imbalances?

Multiple Choice

(546) 42. The best way for the nurse to determine the patient's fluid balance is to:
1. assess vital signs.
2. weigh the patient daily.
3. monitor IV fluid intake.
4. check diagnostic test results.

(547) 43. For the patient with intracellular dehydration, the nurse anticipates that the patient will receive a:
1. hypotonic solution.
2. hypertonic solution.
3. isotonic solution.
4. parenteral feeding.

CHAPTER

22 Mathematics Review and Medication Administration

Answer Key: Textbook page references are provided as a guide for answering these questions. A complete answer key was provided for your instructor.

TERMS

Objective

- Define the key terms as listed.

Match the terms in Column A with the appropriate definition or description in Column B.

Column A			Column B
(604)	1.	_____ Anaphylactic shock	a. One drug increasing the effect of another drug
(585)	2.	_____ Buccal	b. A unique hypersensitivity to a particular drug
(598)	3.	_____ Drip factor	c. Shell that encases a tablet to keep it from being absorbed in the stomach
(581)	4.	_____ Enteric-coated	d. Routes other than digestive system
(574)	5.	_____ Idiosyncratic	e. Applied to the skin
(583)	6.	_____ Meniscus	f. In the cheek
(581)	7.	_____ Parenteral	g. Curve formed by liquid's upper surface
(573)	8.	_____ Potentiation	h. Apparatus used to deliver measured amounts of IV solutions
(585)	9.	_____ Sublingual	i. Under the tongue
(582)	10.	_____ Topical application	j. Severe, life-threatening hypersensitivity

CALCULATION

Objectives

- Confidently use basic mathematical skills to solve dosage problems accurately.
- Set up and work problems using the following formula: (desired dose/available dose) × amount.
- Set up and work problems using the proportion method.
- Use "key" equivalents of metric and apothecary measurement systems in dosage problems.
- Convert measurement units within the metric system.
- Convert between measurement units of the metric system and the apothecary system.
- Determine the appropriateness of dosage orders for children by the use of Young's, Clark's, and Fried's rules and the body surface area.

(564)   11.   For fractions, provide examples of the following:

Numerator _____

Denominator _____

Proper fraction _____

Improper fraction_____

Mixed fraction _____

(564)   12.   Change the following improper fractions to mixed fractions:

$\frac{8}{5} =$ $\frac{100}{13} =$

$\frac{12}{7} =$ $\frac{30}{4} =$

$\frac{7}{6} =$

(564)   13.   Change the following mixed fractions to improper fractions:

$7\frac{5}{8} =$ $9\frac{1}{3} =$

$8\frac{1}{5} =$ $6\frac{5}{7} =$

$15\frac{1}{4} =$

(564)   14.   Reduce the following fractions to their lowest terms:

$\frac{4}{8} =$ $\frac{5000}{1000} =$

$\frac{3}{9} =$ $\frac{8}{40} =$

$\frac{21}{3} =$ $\frac{4}{16} =$

$\frac{15}{30} =$ $\frac{18}{3} =$

$\frac{25}{100} =$ $\frac{75}{50} =$

Student Name_____

(565) 15. Identify which is the largest fraction in the each group:

$^{6}/_{14}$ $^{8}/_{14}$ $^{13}/_{14}$

$^{3}/_{4}$ $^{4}/_{5}$ $^{7}/_{8}$

(565) 16. Add the following fractions and reduce the sum to its lowest term:

$^{1}/_{2} + ^{5}/_{2} + ^{3}/_{2} =$ $\qquad$ $^{2}/_{12} + ^{5}/_{12} + ^{9}/_{12} =$

$^{2}/_{5} + ^{1}/_{3} + ^{7}/_{10} =$ $\qquad$ $2^{1}/_{3} + 5^{1}/_{4} =$

$^{1}/_{3} + ^{1}/_{5} =$

(566) 17. Subtract the following fractions and reduce the answer to its lowest term:

$^{4}/_{5} - ^{1}/_{5} =$ $\qquad$ $^{4}/_{5} - ^{1}/_{7} =$

$^{1}/_{2} - ^{1}/_{3} =$ $\qquad$ $^{3}/_{4} - ^{1}/_{4} =$

$2^{3}/_{4} - 1^{1}/_{2} =$

(566) 18. Multiply the following fractions and reduce the product to its lowest term:

$^{1}/_{3} \times ^{3}/_{12} =$ $\qquad$ $^{2}/_{5} \times ^{1}/_{7} =$

$2^{7}/_{8} \times 3^{1}/_{3} =$ $\qquad$ $41 \times ^{3}/_{4} =$

$^{1}/_{2} \times ^{1}/_{5} =$

(566) 19. Divide the following fractions and reduce the answer to its lowest term:

$^{1}/_{2} \div ^{1}/_{3} =$ $\qquad$ $^{5}/_{3} \div ^{5}/_{3} =$

$2^{1}/_{4} \div ^{1}/_{7} =$ $\qquad$ $^{3}/_{10} \div ^{5}/_{25} =$

$^{5}/_{8} \div ^{3}/_{4} =$

(567) 20. Add the following decimals:

$5.4 + 6.9 =$ $\qquad$ $4.297 + 1.919 =$

$4.25 + 3.217 =$ $\qquad$ $2.2 + 1.68 =$

$22.1 + 0.75 =$

(567)   21. Subtract the following decimals:

$0.089 - 0.0057 =$ $15.6 - 1.2 =$

$2.69 - 1.678 =$ $75.1 - 24.2 =$

$1.5 - 0.22 =$

(567)   22. Round the following decimals to hundredths and then to tenths:

$5.753 =$ $52.371 =$

$4.215 =$ $0.604 =$

$3.178 =$

(567)   23. Multiply the following decimals:

$4.2 \times 5.75 =$ $2.197 \times 0.93 =$

$64.75 \times 22.9 =$ $22.5 \times 50 =$

$33.1 \times 25.95 =$

(568)   24. Divide the following decimals and round to the nearest hundredth:

$5.6 \div 6.97 =$ $0.02 \div 0.0007 =$

$2.9 \div 0.218 =$ $75 \div 2.2 =$

$45.62 \div 1.4 =$

(568)   25. Convert the following fractions into decimals:

$\frac{1}{4} =$ $\frac{3}{4} =$

$\frac{1}{2} =$ $\frac{4}{8} =$

$\frac{1}{5} =$

(568)   26. Convert the following fractions into percents:

$\frac{75}{100} =$ $\frac{5}{10} =$

$\frac{1}{3} =$ $\frac{20}{100} =$

$\frac{42}{100} =$

Student Name_____

(569)   27.   In the following ratios, solve for X:

20 : 40 = X : 5   X =

$^1/_{150}$: 2 = $^1/_{250}$: X   X =

X : 9 = 4 : 12   X =

$^1/_2$: 2 = $^1/_3$: X   X =

X : 1 = 0.4 : 6   X =

(570)   28.   Complete the following equivalents:

30 ml = _____ ounces   400 ml = _____ L

1000 ml = _____ L   2 mcg = _____ mg

1 L = _____ quarts   4 mg = _____ gr

500 ml = _____ pints   44 lb = _____ kg

60 mg = _____ gr   5 mg = _____ mcg

1 kg = _____ pounds

(572)   29.   What are the differences between Young's rule, Clark's rule, and Fried's rule?

(570)   30.   Calculate the patient's total fluid intake for breakfast: 8 ounces of milk, 6 ounces of juice, and 10 ounces of coffee:

_____ cc

(569)   31.   The order is for Tegretol 200 mg po tid.

Available—Tegretol 100 mg tablets.

How many tablets should be given per dose?

(569)   32.   The order is for Aldomet 250 mg po bid.

Available—Aldomet 125 mg tablets.

How many tablets should be given per dose?

(569)   33.   The order is for V-Cillin K suspension 500,000 U po.

Available—V-Cillin K suspension 200,000 U/5 ml.

How much should be prepared?

(569)   34.   The order is for morphine 4 mg IM prn for pain.

Available—morphine 10 mg/ml.

You prepare: _____ ml

(569)   35.   The order is for heparin 5000 U sc.

On hand is heparin 10,000 U/ml.

How much should be given?

(569)   36.   The order is for Solu-Medrol 50 mg IV.

On hand is Solu-Medrol 125 mg/2 ml.

How much is prepared?

(572)   37.   Using Young's rule, identify the dose for a child who is 3 years old and the adult dose is 75 mg.

(572)   38.   Using Clark's rule, identify the dose for a child who weighs 30 lb and the adult dose is 50 mg.

(572)   39.   Using Fried's rule, identify the dose for a child who is 10 months old and the adult dose is 100 mg.

(573)   40.   Using the body surface area calculation, identify the dose for a child with a BSA of 1.1 m^2 and the adult dose is 10 mg.

Student Name _____

Multiple Choice

(571)   41. An order for codeine gr ½ is written for the patient. The medication is supplied in mg. You should administer:

1. 3 g.
2. 30 g.
3. 3 mg.
4. 30 mg.

DRUG ACTION

Objectives

- Explain each phase of drug action.
- Explain the importance of decreased hepatic and renal functioning.

(573)   42. Identify the two general types of drug actions.

(574)   43. Describe possible responses that patients may have to medications.

(575)   44. Provide two examples of how older adults may respond to medications and nursing interventions to prevent their occurrence or reduce their severity.

DRUG DOSAGE

Objectives

- Discuss drug dosage.
- Discuss minimal dosage.
- Discuss maximal dosage.
- Discuss toxic dosage.

- Discuss lethal dosage.
- Discuss potentiation.
- Explain the importance of an antagonist counteracting an agonist.
- Describe five factors that affect drug action in patients.

(573)   45.   What are the terms used to describe drug dosage?

(574)   46.   What factors can influence a patient's response to a medication?

(574)   47.   Provide an example of a drug interaction.

DRUG ORDERS

Objectives

- Describe factors to consider in choosing routes of administration of medication.
- Describe the importance of accurate transcription of medication orders.
- Give the order of priority in the following terms: stat, ASAP, now, and prn.
- Explain what is meant by a controlled substance.
- List three ways medication orders are given.

(576)   48.   What is the difference between the trade name and generic name of a drug?

(576)   49.   A medication order should include:

Student Name_____

(576)   50.   Put the following terms in order of priority:

      prn _____

      now _____

      stat _____

      ASAP _____

(576)   51.   Provide an example of a controlled substance and the special nursing considerations for storage and administration.

(578)   52.   Identify the different types of medication orders.

(579)   53.   Identify the meaning of the following abbreviations:

      bid _____

      tid _____

      qid _____

      pc _____

      hs _____

(581)   54.   Provide an example of a form of medication for each of the following routes:

      Enteral _____

      Percutaneous _____

      Parenteral _____

NURSING

Objectives

- Discuss the nurse's role and responsibilities in medication administration.
- List the "six rights" of drug administration.
- Discuss "Safety Tips from Nurse-Experts."

(579)   55.   What are the "six rights" of medication administration?

(576)   56.   For the following situations, identify what you should do.

The prescriber's handwriting on the medication order sheet is hard to read.

Another nurse asks you to administer to her patient the medications she has prepared.

The dosage of the medication ordered appears high.

(579)   57.   What are some of the guidelines for documentation of medication administration?

(580)   58.   Identify three safety tips for administration of medications.

Student Name _____

(581)   59.   Identify home health safety information that should be included in a teaching plan for medication administration.

(582)   60.   You are preparing to administer oral medications to the patient. How are the following prepared?

Pills from a multidose vial _____

Tablets in unit dose packages _____

(583)   61.   You are preparing to administer a liquid medication to the patient.

What equipment is needed?

How is the liquid poured?

How is the dosage amount checked?

(583)   62.   The site selected for a transdermal patch application should be:

_____.

(584)   63.   Medication is to be administered via a nasogastric tube.

It is critical for the nurse to check: _____.

Equipment needed:

Medication administration is followed by: _____.

(585)   64.   An example of a sublingual medication is: _____.

(585)   65.   For a rectal suppository, the nurse places the patient in _____ position

and prepares the suppository for insertion by: _____.

(587) 66. The nurse is evaluating the patient's administration of eye drops that are ordered i OD. Identify which actions require correction:

The patient touches the tip of the bottle to the eyelid. _____

One drop is administered to the left eye. _____

The drop is placed in the conjunctival sac. _____

(585) 67. In preparing to give ear drops to an adult patient, the nurse will pull the earlobe:

_____.

(587) 68. For the following, identify the type of syringe or needle required:

Administration of 0.25 ml of medication

An IM injection of 1.5 ml of a nonviscous medication to an average-sized adult.

(590) 69. How can needle sticks be prevented?

(591) 70. What information should be included in a teaching plan for a patient who requires a metered-dose inhaler without a spacer?

(592) 71. What sites can be used for a subcutaneous injection?

(593) 72. For a buccal medication, identify which action is correct:

Placing the medication between the cheek and gum. _____

Following the medication with a glass of water. _____

(596) 73. Identify the common medications that are used in patient-controlled analgesia (PCA) and the nurse's responsibilities associated with this administration.

(598) 74. What is the procedure for mixing two medications in one syringe?

Student Name _____

(598)   75. A microdrip IV set is _____ drops/ml.

(601)   76. What are the responsibilities of the nurse in monitoring IV therapy?

(599)   77. An IV is ordered to infuse at 75 ml/hr. The drip factor is 10 gtt/ml. The rate of infusion

should be _____ gtt/min.

(599)   78. An IV is ordered to infuse at 30 ml/hr with a microdrip set. The rate of infusion should be

_____ gtt/min.

(599)   79. An IV of 1000 ml is to infuse over 6 hours. The drip factor is 15 gtt/ml. The rate of

infusion should be _____ gtt/min.

(603)   80. For an IM injection, identify the following:

Angle of insertion _____

Preparation of the site _____

Action to take if blood is returned on aspiration _____

(607)   81. Identify the responsibilities of the nurse in the administration of medications.

(608)   82. What problem does polypharmacy pose for the older adult?

Multiple Choice

(599)   83. An IV of 500 ml D_5W is to infuse over 4 hours. The administration set is 15 gtt/ml. How
many gtt/min should the infusion run?
1.   19
2.   24
3.   31
4.   42

(599)   84.   The nurse determines the location for an injection by identifying the greater trochanter of the femur, anterosuperior iliac spine, and the iliac crest. The injection site being used by the nurse is the:
1.   rectus femoris.
2.   ventrogluteal.
3.   dorsogluteal.
4.   vastus lateralis.

(579)   85.   Upon getting the assignment for the evening, the nurse notices that two patients on the unit have the same last name. The best way to prevent medication errors for these two patients is to:
1.   ask the patients their names.
2.   check the patient's ID bands.
3.   ask another nurse about their identities.
4.   verify their names with the family members.

(591)   86.   The nurse is working in the newborn nursery and will be giving vitamin K injections to the babies. The site preferred for these injections is:
1.   deltoid.
2.   dorsogluteal.
3.   ventrogluteal.
4.   vastus lateralis.

(576)   87.   When preparing a narcotic medication, the nurse drops the pill on the floor. The nurse should:
1.   discard the medication.
2.   notify the pharmacy.
3.   wipe off the medication and administer it.
4.   have another nurse witness the disposal of the pill.

(592)   88.   The Z-track technique is used by the nurse when the patient is:
1.   extremely obese.
2.   less than 5 years old.
3.   receiving an irritating medication.
4.   having a large dosage of medication given.

(605)   89.   A Mantoux skin test will be given to the patient. In selecting the site for this intradermal injection, the nurse assesses the:
1.   upper outer aspect of the arm.
2.   anterior aspect of the forearm.
3.   middle third of the anterior thigh.
4.   2-inch diameter around the umbilicus.

(598)   90.   How does the nurse determine what the drip factor is for an IV set?
1.   Ask the primary nurse.
2.   Calculate the IV rate.
3.   Look in a reference book.
4.   Check the IV tubing box.

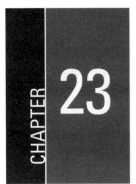

CHAPTER 23

Student Name _____

Emergency First Aid Nursing

Answer Key: Textbook page references are provided as a guide for answering these questions. A complete answer key was provided for your instructor.

TERMS

Objective

- Define the key terms as listed.

    1. Define the following terms:

(620)   Cyanosis _____

(624)   Ecchymosis _____

(622)   Embolism _____

(623)   Epistaxis _____

(626)   Flail chest _____

(623)   Hematemesis _____

(625)   Pneumothorax _____

(619)   Stridor _____

NURSING

Objectives

- List the priorities of assessment to be performed when arriving at a situation requiring first aid.
- Discuss moral, legal, and physical interventions of performing first aid.

(613)   2.   How are the Good Samaritan laws related to emergency situations?

(613)   3.   What is the nursing responsibility in assessment and treatment of a victim in an emergency?

Multiple Choice

(613)   4.   You arrive outside of the public library and find a person lying on the ground. The first action to take is to:
1. check if the victim is unconscious.
2. check the carotid or brachial pulse.
3. move the victim to a flat, hard surface.
4. call to have someone activate the emergency medical system (call 911).

CARDIOPULMONARY RESUSCITATION (CPR)

Objectives

- List the reasons cardiopulmonary resuscitation (CPR) should be performed.
- Discuss the legal implications of CPR.
- List the steps in performing one-rescuer and two-rescuer CPR on the adult victim.
- List the steps in performing CPR on the infant and child.

(614)   5.   When is CPR performed?

(614)   6.   What are the "ABCs" for assessing the emergency patient?

(614)   7.   The nurse opens the patient's airway by:

(616)   8.   What is the rate of mouth-to-mouth ventilation for an adult victim?

(615)   9.   For CPR, identify the following:

Check the pulse at the: _____

If no pulse: _____

Student Name_____

Placement of hands: _____

Depress the sternum for an adult: _____

Ratio of compressions to breaths: _____

(616) 10. Describe the steps for one-rescuer CPR.

(617) 11. For pediatric CPR, if help cannot be obtained right away, the rescuer should:

_____.

(618) 12. For pediatric CPR, identify the following:

	Infant	Child
Where the pulse is checked		
Ratio of compressions/breaths		

Multiple Choice

(615) 13. For CPR to an adult victim, a single rescuer provides breaths at a rate of:
   1. 8 per minute.
   2. 12 per minute.
   3. 20 per minute.
   4. 24 per minute.

AIRWAY

Objectives

• Name the steps in performing the Heimlich maneuver on conscious and unconscious victims.
• Discuss management of airway obstruction in the child and the infant.

(618) 14. For a possible airway obstruction, the victim is coughing. What should you do?

(619)   15. Describe the procedure for the Heimlich maneuver for a conscious adult victim.

What is the difference in the procedure for an unconscious victim?

(620)   16. How is the airway clearance procedure for an infant different?

Multiple Choice

(618)   17. A sign or symptom of a foreign body airway obstruction that requires immediate attention is the:
   1.   ability of the victim to speak.
   2.   ability of the victim to cough forcefully.
   3.   presence of wheezing between coughs.
   4.   presence of a high-pitched inspiratory noise.

(619)   18. When performing the Heimlich maneuver, the fist should be placed:
   1.   over the ribs.
   2.   over the sternum.
   3.   slightly above the navel.
   4.   over the xiphoid process.

(620)   19. For an unconscious adult victim with a foreign body airway obstruction, a nurse should:
   1.   apply a series of three quick chest thrusts.
   2.   repeat chest thrusts continuously 10 times.
   3.   perform finger sweeps between abdominal thrusts.
   4.   attempt to ventilate the victim after each abdominal thrust.

SHOCK

Objectives

- Discuss the signs and symptoms of shock.
- List nursing interventions to treat shock.

Student Name_____

(620)　　　20.　Identify the different types of shock.

(620)　　　21.　What assessments lead the nurse to believe that a victim/patient is in shock?

(621)　　　22.　What are the interventions for a victim/patient who is in shock?

INJURY

Objectives

- Discuss three methods of controlling hemorrhage.
- Define four types of wounds.
- Discuss treatment of wounds.
- Discuss methods of treating three common types of poisonings.
- List the characteristics of assessment of bone, joint, and muscle injuries.
- Discuss emergency care for suspected injuries.

(621)　　　23.　If the victim has a suspected head, neck, or spinal injury, the nurse rescuer should:

(622)　　　24.　What are the effects of blood loss on the body?

(622)   25.   What are the nursing interventions for a victim/patient who is bleeding?

(623)   26.   Epistaxis is fairly common. What are the nursing interventions for an individual experiencing this problem?

(624)   27.   The individual has a closed wound. What are the appropriate nursing interventions?

(625)   28.   Identify the different types of open wounds and an example of a specific nursing intervention for each type.

(626)   29.   The victim had an accident and now has a piece of wood protruding from the chest. The nurse should:

(626)   30.   What interventions should be taken for an individual with a sucking wound to the chest?

Student Name_____

(627)   31. What is the first action to take when there is a suspected poisoning?

(627)   32. For the a victim of a poisoning, identify the assessments that may be made for these body systems:

Respiratory _____

Neurological _____

Gastrointestinal _____

(627)   33. The nurse is instructed to provide water to a poisoning victim to dilute the substance ingested. Identify how much water should be given to an adult and a child.

(627)   34. The nurse is instructed to give syrup of ipecac to a poisoning victim. Identify the amount of ipecac that should be given to an adult and a child.

(628)   35. Vomiting is not induced if an individual has ingested: _____.

(628)   36. An employee has been exposed to a chemical that may be absorbed through the skin. The

nurse should assist by: _____.

(631)   37. After assessing the ABCs in a victim with a bone injury, the nurse should:

_____.

(632)   38. What are the interventions associated with the following acronym?

R _____

I _____

C _____

E _____

(632)   39. Identify areas that should be included in a teaching plan for safety and response to emergency in the home environment.

THERMAL INJURY

Objectives

- Define three types of burns.
- Discuss the nursing interventions in the first aid treatment of burns.
- Describe the nursing interventions of heat and cold emergencies.

(630)   40.   What are the signs and symptoms of heatstroke?

(630)   41.   What are the signs and symptoms of hypothermia?

(633)   42.   Describe the three different types of burns.

(633)   43.   What are the nursing interventions for a patient/victim with a moderate burn?

(634)   44.   An adult patient has severe burns to the thorax and both upper extremities. Using the Rule of Nines, how much of the body surface is burned?

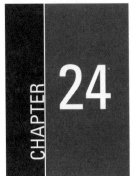

CHAPTER 24

Health Promotion and Pregnancy

Answer Key: Textbook page references are provided as a guide for answering these questions. A complete answer key was provided for your instructor.

TERMS

Objective

- Define the key terms as listed.

  1. Define the following terms:

  (651)   Amniocentesis _____

  (655)   Gravida _____

  (639)   Morula _____

  (655)   Para _____

  (639)   Teratogenic agent _____

PHYSIOLOGY

Objectives

- Explain the physiology of conception.
- Discuss the anatomic and physiologic alterations that occur during pregnancy.

(638)   2. Fertilization occurs in the: _____. The new cell is called the:

        _____.

(639)   3. Enzymes are secreted by the _____ to allow for implantation.

        Implantation occurs in the _____ of the uterus.

(639)   4. The embryonic stage of development lasts for _____ weeks. After this initial stage, the

        embryo is called the: _____.

(650)   5.   What is the role of the placenta?

(640)   6.   Identify the usual time that the following developments occur in the mother or fetus:

Morning sickness _____

Genitalia are defined _____

Swallowing and sucking begin _____

Stretch marks, redness, and darkening of the skin _____

Surfactant forms in the lungs _____

(650)   7.   What is the function of amniotic fluid?

(648)   8.   What maternal antibodies are usually transferred to the fetus?

(651)   9.   What is the highest level of the uterus at full term?

(652)   10.   The usual length of time for an uncomplicated pregnancy is: _____.

This time is divided into: _____.

Multiple Choice

(642)   11.   The woman asks the nurse when the baby's heartbeat can be heard. The nurse responds by saying "The heartbeat can be heard by week _____."
1.   6
2.   8
3.   10
4.   16

Student Name_____

(642)   12.   The very first fetal movements, characterized as "bubbling through a straw" in the stomach, may be experienced at:
1.   4 weeks.
2.   6 weeks.
3.   10 weeks.
4.   18 weeks.

HEALTH ASSESSMENT

Objectives

- Compare the presumptive, possible, and positive signs of pregnancy.
- Discuss the common discomforts of pregnancy.
- List the danger signs that might occur during pregnancy.
- Discuss cultural practices and beliefs that may affect ongoing health care during pregnancy.
- Identify the components of antepartal assessment.

(649)   13.   The mother asks the nurse why she is having such terrible backaches. The nurse responds by telling the woman that:

(653)   14.   A basic prenatal exam usually includes:

(653)   15.   What aspects are important in genetic counseling?

(653)   16.   An obstetrical assessment should include information on the patient's:

(654)   17. In determination of pregnancy, identify the following:

Presumptive signs _____

Probable signs _____

Positive signs _____

(655)   18. The patient had her last menstrual period (LMP) on August 18. Using Nagele's rule, when is the estimated date of birth (EDB)?

(650)   19. What is the usual preparation for an ultrasound?

(651)   20. What tests are used to determine the well-being of the fetus?

(656)   21. Define the parity of the following woman using the GTPAL system:

She has been pregnant four times, delivered three full-term infants, had no abortions or preterm deliveries, and has three living children.

(658)   22. Describe some of the common skin changes that occur during pregnancy.

Student Name _____

(662) 23. Psychological aspects that should be considered during the pregnancy are:

Multiple Choice

(654) 24. The patient believes that she is pregnant. On examination, Chadwick's sign is found. This is:
1. a sensation of fetal movement.
2. softening of the cervix.
3. darkened pigmentation of the cheeks.
4. purplish discoloration of the vagina, vulva, and cervix.

(652) 25. An early amniocentesis is performed to determine:
1. fetal distress.
2. fetal lung maturity.
3. presence of intrauterine infection.
4. presence of biochemical abnormalities.

NURSING

Objectives

- Describe nutritional requirements during pregnancy.
- Identify nursing diagnoses relevant to care of the prenatal patient.

(640) 26. What interventions are appropriate for the following maternal discomforts?

Morning sickness _____

Headaches _____

Leg cramps _____

Indigestion _____

(640) 27. Identify five drugs that the mother should avoid during pregnancy.

(656) 28. Identify the areas of counseling for self-care on the trimester checklist.

(657) 29. What signs and symptoms should the nurse instruct the woman to report during the pregnancy?

(657) 30. The nurse instructs the woman to avoid the following during the pregnancy:

(658) 31. For the following systems, identify common problems that may develop during pregnancy and interventions to relieve them:

Gastrointestinal _____

Urinary _____

(659) 32. Identify two common discomforts experienced during the third trimester and the teaching for self-care for each one.

(660) 33. The usual position of comfort for the woman to sleep or rest is:

_____.

(660) 34. What counseling is appropriate regarding sexual activity for the pregnant woman?

(663) 35. Identify an example of a cultural or ethnic consideration for pregnancy.

Student Name _____

(665) 36. Identify general prenatal nursing interventions.

(664) 37. Formulate a nursing diagnosis, patient outcome, and nursing interventions for a woman experiencing a nonrisk pregnancy.

Multiple Choice

(657) 38. The nurse informs the patient to report which of the following during the pregnancy?
1. reddened palms
2. urinary frequency
3. swelling of the face
4. dilated capillaries on the skin

(658) 39. The patient asks the nurse what can be done specifically about the ptyalism that the physician told her about. The nurse instructs the patient to:
1. eat small, frequent meals.
2. suck on hard candy.
3. sit up after eating.
4. avoid eating spicy foods.

(661) 40. Which of the following should be included in a plan for prenatal exercise?
1. Exercise one time per week.
2. Exercise for 30 minutes, then rest.
3. Keep moving after exercising.
4. Reduce exercise sharply 4 weeks before the due date.

Student Name _____

Labor and Delivery

Answer Key: Textbook page references are provided as a guide for answering these questions. A complete answer key was provided for your instructor.

TERMS

Objective

- Define the key terms as listed.

Match the terms in Column A with the appropriate definition or description in Column B.

	Column A		Column B
(668)	1. _____ Braxton-Hicks contractions	a.	Part that first enters the pelvis and lies over the inlet
(668)	2. _____ Effacement	b.	Insufficient availability of oxygen to meet metabolic needs
(681)	3. _____ Episiotomy	c.	Hormone produced by the pituitary gland.
(681)	4. _____ Expulsion	d.	First stools of the infant
(671)	5. _____ Fetal presentation	e.	Irregular tightening of the pregnant uterus that begins in the first trimester
(677)	6. _____ Hypoxia	f.	Thinning and shortening of the cervix
(667)	7. _____ Lightening	g.	Midline incision in which the tissues of the perineum are separated
(677)	8. _____ Meconium	h.	Fetus seems to have settled or "dropped" into the pelvis
(683)	9. _____ Oxytocin	i.	Head moves to realign with the body and shoulders
(681)	10. _____ Restitution	j.	Body of the infant leaves the pelvis

IMPENDING LABOR

Objectives

- Explain the five factors that affect the labor process.
- Discuss the signs and symptoms of impending labor.
- Distinguish between true and false labor.

(667)   11.   Identify the signs of impending labor.

(668)   12.   Provide a few examples of true versus false labor.

(668)   13.   The woman is asking about delivering somewhere other than a hospital. The nurse provides the following information:

PROCESS OF LABOR AND DELIVERY

Objectives

- Discuss fetopelvic disproportion.
- Describe the "powers" involved in labor and delivery.
- Identify the mechanisms of labor.
- Identify the stages of labor.

(669)   14.   The 5 'P's of labor are:

(669)   15.   What influence does the passageway have on labor and delivery?

Student Name _____

(671)   16.   What is meant by each of the following?

Fetal attitude _____

Fetal lie _____

Fetal presentation _____

Fetal position _____

(672)   17.   How is the position of the fetus determined?

(672)   18.   Identify what the following abbreviations indicate:

ROP _____

LOA _____

LSA _____

(674)   19.   What is the normal fetal heart rate? _____

What do the following changes in fetal heart rate indicate?

Late deceleration _____

Variable deceleration _____

(677)   20.   What signs precede the delivery of the placenta and what is done after the delivery of the placenta?

(678)   21.   What is the usual frequency and duration of uterine contractions and what is their purpose?

(680)   22.   What position(s) are most effective for delivery?

(680)   23.   Provide a brief overview of the steps in the process of labor.

Multiple Choice

(681)   24.   On examination, the patient is found to be 8 cm dilated with contractions every 3 minutes that last for 70 seconds. She also does not want to communicate with the nurse or her coach. This is point in labor is described as:
1.   early latent phase.
2.   mid/active phase.
3.   transitional phase.
4.   second stage.

(681)   25.   A woman who is in the mid/active phase of labor will be expected to have:
1.   2 cm cervical dilation.
2.   contractions every 4 minutes.
3.   a desire to ambulate.
4.   very mild, easily controlled pain.

(681)   26.   The second stage of labor begins at the:
1.   onset of contractions.
2.   rupture of the amniotic sac.
3.   dilation of the cervix to 10 cm.
4.   delivery of the placenta.

(696)   27.   When coaching the patient through the early/latent phase of labor, the nurse uses the breathing technique of:
1.   shallow panting.
2.   slow, deep chest or abdominal breathing.
3.   acceleration through contractions.
4.   holding the breath for 5 seconds and exhaling.

INTERVENTIONS—NURSING AND MEDICAL

Objectives

- Describe the assessment for labor and delivery.
- Explain breathing techniques beneficial for the patient in labor.
- Identify nursing diagnoses relevant to the woman in labor.
- Outline medical interventions related to labor and delivery.
- Discuss nursing interventions related to labor and delivery.

Student Name_____

(688)   28.   The admission assessment to the labor area includes:

(672)   29.   How is fetal status monitored?

(677)   30.   The nurse suspects fetal distress because of the presence of:

(689)   31.   The monitor indicates a late deceleration. The patient is positioned:

(677)   32.   Identify the interventions for a prolapsed cord.

(693)   33.   For regional anesthesia during labor, what are the possible effects on the fetus and appropriate nursing interventions?

(690)   34. The nurse's response to the husband or coach is very important. How can the nurse provide a positive experience for the mother's support person?

(694)   35. Nursing assessment of a patient's status throughout labor includes:

(696)   36. What is the goal of the breathing techniques that are used throughout labor?

(696)   37. Medical intervention during labor includes induction. Why is this implemented and what methods are used?

(694)   38. Identify two nursing diagnoses for a woman in labor.

(697)   39. Identify a nursing diagnosis for a woman who has had a cesarean delivery.

Student Name_____

(681)   40.   What is the purpose of an episiotomy?

(684)   41.   For the fourth stage of labor, what are the nursing assessments and how often are they done?

(685)   42.   Provide at least one example of a medication commonly used for pain relief during labor, possible side effects, and nursing interventions.

(687)   43.   The baby is assessed after birth and the following are noted: heart rate—124/minute; respiratory effort good, crying; some flexion of the extremities; grimacing; body pink, extremities bluish.

Based on this information, what is the Apgar score?

(687)   44.   Care of the baby after birth includes:

(692)   45.   Complications of a precipitous labor are:

Multiple Choice

(689)   46.   The nurse recognizes that which of the following is an acceptable practice in labor and delivery?
1.   maintenance of a full bladder
2.   maintenance of supine position
3.   ambulation prior to membrane rupture
4.   administration of enemas to a patient with vaginal bleeding

(697)   47.   The patient is receiving IV pitocin for the stimulation of labor. The nurse identifies that the fetal heart rate (FHR) is dropping below 100/min. The nurse should:
1.   stop the infusion.
2.   slow down the infusion.
3.   monitor the FHR for 5–10 full cycles of contractions.
4.   do nothing as this is an expected response.

CHAPTER 26

Student Name _____

Care of the Mother and Newborn

Answer Key: Textbook page references are provided as a guide for answering these questions. A complete answer key was provided for your instructor.

TERMS

Objective

- Define the key terms as listed.

Match the terms in Column A with the appropriate definition or description in Column B.

		Column A		Column B
(722)	1.	_____ Acrocyanosis	a.	Downy, fine hair
(724)	2.	_____ Cryptorchidism	b.	Decrease in uterine size
(713)	3.	_____ Engorgement	c.	Vaginal discharge during puerperium of blood, tissue, and mucus
(722)	4.	_____ Fontanelle	d.	Extra digits
(722)	5.	_____ Harlequin sign	e.	Uncomfortable fullness of the breasts when milk supply comes in
(701)	6.	_____ Involution	f.	Hands and feet appear slightly blue
(722)	7.	_____ Lanugo	g.	Half of the body appears deep red and the other side pale
(701)	8.	_____ Lochia	h.	Broad area or soft spot located at the junction of the bones
(724)	9.	_____ Polydactyly	i.	Yellowish-white, cream cheese-like substance
(722)	10.	_____ Vernix caseosa	j.	Undescended testicles

POSTPARTUM

Objectives

- Describe postpartum assessment of the mother.
- Identify the physiologic changes that occur in the postpartum period.
- Discuss the psychosocial adaptations that occur postpartum.
- Explain parent-child attachment (bonding).

(701)   11. Identify the height of the fundus through the process of involution:

Immediately after delivery _____

12 hours after delivery _____

24–48 hours after delivery _____

1 week after delivery _____

6 weeks after delivery _____

(701)   12. Identify the types of lochia and the characteristics from delivery through the first 14 days after delivery.

(702)   13. What type of nonlochia bleeding should be reported right away?

(702)   14. What processes are involved in lactation?

(702)   15. Identify the changes that occur in the following body systems after delivery:

Cardiovascular _____

Urinary _____

Gastrointestinal _____

Endocrine _____

Integumentary _____

(704)   16. Identify postpartum danger signs:

Physical _____

Parent-child _____

Student Name _____

(705)   17.   What are the basic nutritional needs of the postpartum patient?

(708)   18.   For hygienic care:

         Women following a vaginal delivery should avoid: _____.

         Women following a cesarean delivery should avoid: _____.

(711)   19.   A slight temperature within 24 hours of delivery is usually indicative of:

         _____.

(711)   20.   After delivery, the mother's sleep and rest is usually disturbed by:

         _____.

(720)   21.   Provide an example of a specific cultural practice during the postpartum period.

NEWBORN

Objectives

- Describe the assessment of the normal newborn.
- Identify the physical characteristics of the normal newborn.
- Identify normal reflexes observed in the newborn.
- Explain common variations that may be observed in the newborn.
- Describe the behavioral characteristics of the newborn.
- Discuss nutritional needs and feeding of the newborn.

(721)   22.   For newborn assessment:

         Relationship of head to chest circumference _____

         Temperature _____

         Pulse _____

         Respirations _____

         Blood pressure _____

(722) 23. Indicate for the following assessment findings whether they are expected (normal) or unexpected:

Acrocyanosis within the first 7 days _____

Jaundice within the first 24 hours _____

Lanugo _____

Milia _____

Nevus flammeus _____

Palpable posterior fontanelle _____

Low-set ears _____

Epstein's pearls _____

Molding _____

Two-vessel umbilical cord _____

Syndactyly _____

Gynecomastia _____

Asymmetric popliteal folds _____

(725) 24. Identify some of the important safety measures that should be implemented when working with a newborn.

25. Match the terms in Column A with the appropriate definition or description in Column B.

Column A		**Column B**
(725)	_____ Moro reflex	a. Toes fan out with stroking of the foot.
(725)	_____ Tonic neck reflex	b. Trunk is flexed and pelvis swings to the side where the spine is stimulated.
(725)	_____ Babinski reflex	c. Change in equilibrium causes flexion and abduction of the extremities.
(725)	_____ Galant reflex	d. Arm and leg extend on side of the body that the head is turned toward.

Student Name _____

(729)   26. What are the daily nutritional and fluid needs of the infant?

(730)   27. For feeding the newborn:

What should be done if the baby is allergic to a milk-based formula?

What is the purpose of burping the baby?

(730)   28. How can the nurse reduce the heat loss in a newborn?

(732)   29. Urine and bowel elimination is expected in the newborn within _____ of the delivery.

(732)   30. Identify the characteristics of the newborn's bowel elimination.

Meconium _____

Transitional _____

Breastfed _____

Abnormal _____

(732)   31. Most newborns sleep _____ hours each day.

(732)   32. What is the infant's form of communication?

Multiple Choice

(708)   33. The nurse identifies that the mother requires additional teaching if, for the care of the umbilicus, she:
1.   gives a tub bath in the first 3 days after delivery.
2.   uses alcohol on the stump daily.
3.   folds the diaper down from the umbilicus.
4.   reports a foul odor or redness from the stump.

(708)   34.   Care of the circumcision includes:
1.   removing the yellow crusting right away.
2.   fan-folding the diaper.
3.   applying alcohol to the area.
4.   using petroleum gauze under the Plastibell.

(707)   35.   An appropriate technique to teach the new mother about the baby's bath is:
1.   vigorous removal of the vernix caseosa.
2.   use of plain water on the perineal area.
3.   washing the baby twice daily.
4.   having the bath water at 100° F.

NURSING

Objectives

- Discuss the nursing responsibilities during the postpartum period.
- Explain the importance of teaching personal and infant care.
- Discuss nursing interventions for the circumcised newborn.

(702)   36.   The nurse assesses the episiotomy for:

(711)   37.   Before checking the fundus, the nurse asks the patient to: _____.

(710)   38.   Prior to ambulating a patient for the first time after delivery, the nurse should:

(712)   39.   What types of medications are given to the mother and newborn in the postpartum period?

(714)   40.   How can the nurse assess the amount of lochia?

(714)   41.   Engorgement is treated as follows:

Breastfeeding mother _____

Nonbreastfeeding mother _____

Student Name_____

(715) 42. The patient asks the nurse if breastfeeding is really better for the baby. The nurse informs the patient that the benefits of breastfeeding are:

(717) 43. What does the acronym BUBBLE-HE for postpartum assessment mean?

(716) 44. In the recovery period, assessment of the fundus:

Technique for cesarean delivery _____

Atony is noted _____

(717) 45. The emotional state of the mother changes in the postpartum period. What are the phases that many women go through?

(717) 46. What assessment findings would lead the nurse to believe that the patient is having postpartum emotional problems?

(718) 47. Identify two nursing diagnoses for the postpartum patient.

(733)   48. What behaviors, if observed by the nurse, indicate that the parents are bonding with the infant?

Multiple Choice

(706)   49. The nurse is discussing sexuality with the new mother. Appropriate information to provide is that:
1.   menses usually return in 3–5 months.
2.   breastfeeding acts as an effective contraceptive.
3.   ongoing discomfort and bleeding is expected with sexual activity.
4.   resumption of sexual activity should wait until after the first postpartum office visit.

(707)   50. In teaching the patient about breastfeeding, the nurse informs the mother to:
1.   use only one breast during each feeding.
2.   have the baby nurse for 5 minutes.
3.   put as much of the areolar tissue into the baby's mouth as possible.
4.   pull the breast straight away from the baby's mouth to break the suction seal.

(707)   51. The nurse is teaching the patient about what signs and symptoms should be reported to the health care provider. The patient is instructed to notify the physician if, after 5 days from the delivery date, the patient experiences:
1.   a temperature of 99° F.
2.   lochia that is light pink-brown in color.
3.   breast tenderness and redness.
4.   a fundus that feels like a softball.

Student Name _____

Care of the High-Risk Mother and Newborn

Answer Key: Textbook page references are provided as a guide for answering these questions. A complete answer key was provided for your instructor.

TERMS

Objective

• Define the key terms as listed.

    1.   Define the following terms:

(743)   Cerclage _____

(766)   Erythroblastosis fetalis _____

(747)   Hydramnios _____

(766)   Kernicterus _____

(753)   TORCH _____

HIGH-RISK PREGNANCY

Objectives

• List those conditions that increase maternal and fetal risk.
• Discuss bleeding disorders that can occur during pregnancy.
• Identify diagnostic tests used to determine high-risk situations.
• Describe the HELLP syndrome.
• Discuss pregnancy-induced hypertension.
• Identify preexisting maternal health conditions that influence pregnancy.
• List the infectious disease most likely to cause serious complications.
• Discuss the care of the pregnant adolescent.

(737)   2.   Identify examples of high-risk factors in pregnancy for the following areas:

          Biophysical _____

          Psychosocial _____

Sociodemographic _____

Environmental _____

(738)   3.   Identify factors that place the postpartum mother and infant at risk.

(738)   4.   For hyperemesis gravidarum, identify the signs and symptoms, medical treatment, and nursing interventions:

Signs/symptoms _____

Medical treatment _____

Nursing interventions _____

(739)   5.   The mother has just had twins, a boy and a girl. This is the result of the fertilization of

_____. The term for this is: _____.

(739)   6.   What are the maternal and fetal risks in a multifetal pregnancy?

(740)   7.   Assessment of the presence of a hydatidiform mole is based on:

(741)   8.   Ninety-five percent of ectopic pregnancies occur in the _____.

(741)   9.   For an ectopic pregnancy, identify the signs and symptoms, medical treatment, and nursing interventions:

Signs/symptoms _____

Medical treatment _____

Nursing interventions _____

Student Name_____

(742)   10.   A spontaneous abortion may be the result of:

(742)   11.   The nurse instructs the patient on the treatment for a threatened abortion which includes:

(743)   12.   Treatment for an incompetent cervix usually includes:

(744)   13.   Diagnosis of placenta previa is made when the patient exhibits:

The nurse instructs the patient to expect that treatment for placenta previa may include:

(745)   14.   Medical management of abruptio placentae includes:

(748)   15.   What are the classic signs and symptoms of pregnancy-induced hypertension (PIH)?

(750)   16.   Medical management and nursing interventions for PIH usually include:

(747)   17.   The nurse is assessing the postpartum patient and suspects a hemorrhage as a result of observing:

Treatment for postpartum hemorrhage includes:

(746)   18.   What signs and symptoms may be exhibited by the patient who is experiencing disseminated intravascular coagulation (DIC)?

What diagnostic tests are usually performed to determine the presence of DIC?

(752)   19.   In HELLP syndrome, what happens to the platelet, AST, and ALT levels?

What is a priority of care for a patient with HELLP?

(755)   20.   What complications should the nurse be alert for when the mother is experiencing gestational diabetes?

Student Name _____

(756)   21. The patient with gestational diabetes should anticipate that the following diagnostic tests may be performed:

(760)   22. Postpartum care of the adolescent mother focuses on:

(761)   23. A 45-year-old woman is pregnant. She wants the nurse to tell her what complications of pregnancy are more common for women of her age and if the baby is at risk. The nurse recognizes that the risks for an older woman during pregnancy are:

Multiple Choice

(742)   24. The patient being seen in the obstetrician's office has a missed abortion. The nurse recognizes that this means the patient will have:
1. malodorous bleeding, increased temperature, and cramping.
2. expelled some, but not all, of the products of conception.
3. fetal death and cessation of uterine growth.
4. increased bleeding and a rupture of membranes.

(738)   25. The nurse identifies that the most appropriate outcome for a woman experiencing hyperemesis gravidarum is:
1. relief of painful uterine contractions.
2. absence of fetal withdrawal symptoms.
3. platelets and PT/PTT values within normal limits.
4. adequate caloric intake for maternal and fetal health.

(744)   26. The difference in the diagnosis of placenta previa and abruptio placentae is that abruptio placentae is associated with:
1. decreased vaginal bleeding.
2. sudden uterine pain and rigidity
3. occurrence before 20 weeks gestation.
4. decreased uterine size and poor contractions.

HIGH-RISK NEWBORN

Objectives

- Discuss the problems created by alcohol and drug abuse.
- Identify concerns related to preterm infants.
- Explain the hemolytic disease of the newborn.

(754)   27.   How can the AIDS virus affect the fetus?

(762)   28.   What are the characteristic physical manifestations of a preterm infant?

(764)   29.   Signs and symptoms of newborn respiratory distress include:

Treatment for respiratory distress includes:

(765)   30.   What is a problem seen in infants who are small for gestational age (SGA)?

(765)   31.   Hemolytic disease occurs when:

(765)   32.   Diagnostic tests that are used to determine possible hemolytic disease are:

Student Name_____

(768)　33.　Fetal alcohol syndrome (FAS) may result in the newborn experiencing withdrawal symptoms. The nurse will observe for:

Multiple Choice

(765)　34.　The nurse recognizes that the chance of a hemolytic disease in the newborn is very low if which of the following findings are present?
　　1.　mother blood type O, infant blood type A
　　2.　mother Rh negative, father Rh negative
　　3.　mother Rh negative, infant Rh positive
　　4.　mother blood type B, infant blood type A

NURSING

Objective

- Discuss nursing diagnoses related to high-risk conditions of the mother and newborn.

(745)　35.　Identify the nursing assessment that should take place if the patient experiences bleeding during the pregnancy:

　　36.　Identify possible nursing diagnoses for patients experiencing:

(746)　Abruptio placentae _____

(748)　Postpartum hemorrhage _____

(757)　Gestational diabetes _____

(755)　37.　What teaching should be done about the prevention of an infection during pregnancy?

(758)　38.　What interventions are planned by the nurse for a pregnant patient with a preexisting cardiac condition?

(759)   39. Identify a nursing diagnosis that may be formulated for an adolescent patient during her first experience in labor and delivery.

(764)   40. General nursing interventions for preterm infants include:

(765)   41. Identify a nursing diagnosis that may be formulated for a preterm infant.

Multiple Choice

(748)   42. The nurse is alert to a significant sign of pregnancy-induced hypertension (PIH) which is:
1.   edema.
2.   bradycardia.
3.   weight loss.
4.   hypoglycemia.

(748)   43. The nurse anticipates that the medication to be given to the patient who is experiencing severe PIH will be:
1.   Demerol.
2.   heparin.
3.   oxytocin.
4.   magnesium sulfate.

(760)   44. The nurse is working with an adolescent mother with her first child. A nursing diagnosis that is formulated for this patient is:
1.   Knowledge deficit.
2.   Fluid volume deficit.
3.   Ineffective parenting.
4.   Cardiac output, decreased.

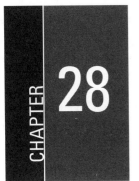

CHAPTER 28

Health Promotion for the Infant, Child, and Adolescent

Answer Key: Textbook page references are provided as a guide for answering these questions. A complete answer key was provided for your instructor.

TERMS

Objective

- Define the key terms as listed.

    1. Define the following terms:

(772) Anticipatory guidance _____

(778) Botulism _____

(778) Nursing bottle caries _____

(779) Syrup of ipecac _____

HEALTH PROMOTION

Objectives

- Identify the 10 "Leading Health Indicators" cited in *Healthy People 2010*.
- List three benefits of regular physical activity in children.
- State American Academy of Pediatrics recommendations for immunization administration in healthy infants and children.
- State three strategies to promote dental health.
- Identify six health benefits associated with exercise, activity, and sports.

(772) 2. Identify the "Leading Health Indicators" from *Healthy People 2010*.

(773)   3.   What are the target goals for the following health indicators?

Physical activity _____

Substance abuse _____

Responsible sexual activity _____

Immunizations _____

(772)   4.   What are the benefits of physical activity?

(773)   5.   How can the nurse promote physical activity for children?

(774)   6.   What factors contribute to obesity in children and adolescents?

(773)   7.   The single most preventable cause of death and disease in the U.S. is:

_____.

(774)   8.   Identify problems associated with substance abuse:

(774)   9.   What information should be taught about responsible sexual behavior?

Student Name _____

(777)   10.   What is the newest guideline regarding immunization for children age 2–23 months?

(778)   11.   Identify strategies to promote dental health for the following age groups:

Infant _____

Preschooler _____

Adolescent _____

SAFETY MEASURES

Objectives

- State the causes and prevention of accidental poisonings.
- Describe four strategies to prevent aspiration of a foreign body.
- Discuss the proper use of infant safety seats in motor vehicles.
- List 10 safety precautions important in educating parents to prevent environmental injuries to children.

(775)   12.   Identify measures to be taken for vehicular safety:

(780)   13.   What strategies may be implemented to prevent accidental poisoning?

(780)   14.   Identify at least five strategies that may be implemented to prevent burns:

(779)   15. For the nursing diagnosis *Poisoning, risk for, related to lack of knowledge of safeguards*, identify at least three interventions or areas for teaching:

(780)   16. Identify strategies that may be implemented to prevent foreign body aspiration.

Multiple Choice

(780)   17. Of the following, which age group is most at risk for foreign body aspiration?
1. 1–5 months
2. 6–12 months
3. 1–2 years
4. 2–4 years

Student Name _____

29 Basic Pediatric Nursing Care

Answer Key: Textbook page references are provided as a guide for answering these questions. A complete answer key was provided for your instructor.

TERMS

Objective

- Define the key terms as listed.

    1.   Define the following terms:

(784)   Birth defect _____

(791)   En face position _____

(782)   Mortality _____

(794)   Weaning _____

HISTORICAL EVENTS

Objectives

- Identify events that had a significant impact on the health care of children in the United States in the twentieth century.
- Discuss the works of Dr. Abraham Jacobi and Lillian Wald.
- Describe the purposes and outcomes of the White House Conference on Children from 1901 to the 1980s.

    2.   Identify the activities associated with the following people or events and the impact upon the development of pediatric care:

(782)   Dr. Abraham Jacobi

(783)   Lillian Wald

(783)   President Theodore Roosevelt (1909)

(783)   President Franklin Roosevelt (1937)

(783)   President Ronald Reagan (1987)

ROLE OF THE PEDIATRIC NURSE

Objectives

- Discuss the personal characteristics and professional skills of a pediatric nurse.
- Identify key elements of family-centered care.
- Describe areas in which growth and development principles are used by the pediatric nurse.

(783)   3.   Identify the main purpose of pediatric nursing.

(784)   4.   What are the characteristics and role of a pediatric nurse?

Student Name _____

(785)   5.   Identify the key elements in family-centered care:

(786)   6.   How are the principles of growth and development used by the nurse?

ASSESSMENT

Objectives

- Discuss the physical assessment of a child using the head-to-toe method.
- Describe metabolism and relationship with nutrition in the child.

(787)   7.   Identify the guidelines for performing a physical assessment on a child:

(790)   8.   The temperature of a 6-month-old is higher _____ or lower _____ than the temperature of an adolescent.

(791)   9.   How does the vision of a child change from infancy to preschool age?

(792)   10.   The nurse is teaching the parents about the development of teeth. The nurse instructs the parents that there are _____(number) of primary teeth that are usually all in place by the age of _____ years. The permanent teeth usually appear by age _____.

(792)   11.   The nurse is preparing to auscultate the child's lungs. Describe methods that can be used to have the child assist in this procedure.

(792)   12.   What spinal abnormalities may be found on an assessment of a child or adolescent?

(793)   13.   What is the usual specific gravity of the child's urine?

                    What is the usual urinary output for a 6-month-old?

(794)   14.   Identify the average time frame for the following foods or nutritional activities to be introduced:

                    Whole milk _____

                    Solid foods (cereals) _____

                    Fruits/vegetables _____

                    Table food _____

                    Weaning _____

(795)   15.   Energy requirements for an infant are highest during _____.

Multiple Choice

(789)   16.   The nurse knows that when assessing the child, the expected annual rate of growth for a 4-year-old is:
           1.   18–22 cm.
           2.   14–18 cm.
           3.   8 cm.
           4.   5 cm.

(789)   17.   The temperature site of choice for an infant is:
           1.   oral.
           2.   rectal.
           3.   tympanic.
           4.   axillary.

(790)   18.   When measuring the vital signs of a 2-year-old, the nurse expects that they will be close to the average findings for that age, which are:
           1.   P 110, R 25, BP 94/66.
           2.   P 100, R 20, BP 110/80.
           3.   P 90, R 22, BP 108/70.
           4.   P 70, R 24, BP 120/76.

Student Name_____

(796)   19. It is expected that the vocabulary for a preschooler will be:
1. 3 or 4 familiar words.
2. 25–50 words.
3. more than 250 words.
4. full, complete sentences.

NURSING INTERVENTIONS

Objectives

- List general strategies to consider when talking with children.
- Outline several approaches for making the hospitalization of children a positive experience for them and their families.
- Discuss pain management in infants and children.
- Explain the needs of parents during their child's hospitalization.
- Discuss common pediatric procedures.
- Discuss administration of pediatric medications.
- Identify each category of age/behavior, accident/hazard, and prevention in the pediatric child.

(790)   20. Describe how you will explain the sensations of blood pressure measurement to a child.

(796)   21. Identify strategies that should be used when communicating with children.

(798)   22. What should the nurse do to reduce anxiety for the child and the parents when the child is admitted to the hospital?

(800)   23. Identify an example of an age-related concern/need of a hospitalized child, the child's possible response, and the positive parent or nurse responses.

Concern/need _____

Child's response _____

Parent/nurse response _____

(799)   24.   Pain is often underestimated in children. What can the nurse do to better assess the child's pain?

(801)   25.   What methods in addition to pain medication can be used for relief or reduction of the child's pain?

(803)   26.   How can the nurse increase the trust and participation of the parents in the care of the hospitalized child?

(803)   27.   The recommended approach for preparing children for procedures is to:

            _____.

            When is it best to prepare younger children for a procedure?

(803)   28.   The nurse is evaluating the bath given to the infant by the adult caregiver. Identify what actions require additional teaching:

            Using soap around the eyes _____

            Using a cotton-tipped swab to clean the ear canal _____

            Supporting the head while bathing the infant in a tub _____

            Washing the extremities after washing the face _____

(805)   29.   How is gavage feeding for the infant provided?

Student Name_____

(806)   30. What are the different types of safety reminder devices that are used for children?

(807)   31. How can urine be collected from an infant?

(808)   32. Following a lumbar puncture, what should the nurse do for the:

Young child_____

Adolescent _____

(808)   33. Delivery of oxygen to a small infant is best provided with:

(809)   34. What assessment findings by the nurse would require the child's airway to be suctioned?

(810)   35. When suctioning a child, the nurse should:

Set wall suction pressure at: _____

Insert the tubing: _____

Suction for: _____ seconds

Suction no more frequently than every: _____

(810)   36. When monitoring intake and output for a child who is not toilet trained, how is the urinary output measured?

(810)   37. What can the nurse offer that will increase the fluid intake and provide variety for the child?

(811)   38. The nurse is to administer an IM injection to a 10-year-old patient. Identify the following:

Site(s) to use: _____

Needle selection: _____

Pain reduction: _____

(813)   39.   What IV site is used for children under 9 months of age?

(813)   40.   For enema administration to children, identify the following:

	Amount	**Tube insertion**
2–4 years old		
11 years old		

Type of solution to use for children: _____

(814)   41.   Provide examples of behaviors, accidents/hazards, and preventive measures from at least two different age groups.

Multiple Choice

(801)   42.   An older school-age child will be having surgery with anesthesia. The nurse intervenes to reduce anxiety by:
1.   showing the child the mask that will be used for the anesthesia.
2.   introducing the child to a peer and having them discuss the procedure.
3.   reassuring the child that only the procedure that is supposed to be done will be completed.
4.   explaining the special type of sleep that will occur with the anesthetic.

(804)   43.   The nurse is discussing nutritional needs of the toddler with his mother. She asks the nurse how to get him to eat right. The nurse responds appropriately by telling the mother that:
1.   food should be left around the house where the child can pick it up when he feels like it.
2.   the child should be restrained in the high chair for meals.
3.   the child should sit at the table for scheduled meals.
4.   meals should be arranged about every 5 hours for the child.

(810)   44.   A medication is to be administered to a child who has a body surface area (BSA) of 0.94 m². The recommended adult dose is 10–20 mg. What is the dosage range that is safe for this child?
1.   5.5 mg–11 mg
2.   9.4 mg–18.8 mg
3.   10 mg–20 mg
4.   11 mg–22 mg

CHAPTER 30

Care of the Child with a Physical Disorder

Answer Key: Textbook page references are provided as a guide for answering these questions. A complete answer key was provided for your instructor.

TERMS

Objective

• Define the key terms as listed.

Match the terms in Column A with the appropriate definition or description in Column B.

	Column A		Column B
(887)	1. _____ Amblyopia	a.	Procedure that involves wrapping the fundus of the stomach around the distal esophagus to prevent reflux
(874)	2. _____ Chelation therapy	b.	Lazy eye; reduction or dimness of vision
(865)	3. _____ Gowers' sign	c.	Partial dislocation
(861)	4. _____ Legg-Calvé-Perthes disease	d.	Persistent penile erection
		e.	Pain and stiffness in the neck when flexed
(876)	5. _____ Lichenification	f.	Use of a compound to grasp a toxic substance and make it nonactive
(850)	6. _____ Nissen fundoplication	g.	Skin becomes thick and leatherlike
(866)	7. _____ Nuchal rigidity	h.	Rising to a standing position by using the hands to "walk up the thighs"
(873)	8. _____ Pica	i.	Caused by decreased blood supply to the femoral head
(828)	9. _____ Priapism	j.	Craving to eat nonfood substances
(860)	10. _____ Subluxation		

CARDIOVASCULAR—HEMATOLOGIC—IMMUNE SYSTEM

Objective

- Discuss the nursing interventions for an infant or a child with congenital heart disease.

(821) 11. Identify the four categories of congenital heart disease and an example of a disorder from each category.

(821) 12. What are the general clinical manifestations of congenital heart disease?

(823) 13. Identify two nursing diagnoses for a child with congenital heart disease.

(825) 14. What are the four defects found in Tetralogy of Fallot?

(825) 15. Identify the clinical signs and symptoms associated with Tetralogy and Fallot and the medical management for the disorder.

(826) 16. The child has a coarctation of the aorta. The nurse expects that the blood pressure measurement will be:

Student Name_____

(827)   17. For the following children, identify the signs and symptoms that may be manifested:

Child with a Hgb of 8 g/dl

Child with a Hgb of 4.8 g/dl

(827)   18. What information should be provided to the parents of the child who is to receive a liquid iron supplement?

(828)   19. Identify an example of a type of sickle cell crisis and the treatment that should be implemented.

(828)   20. Children who have hemophilia and idiopathic thrombocytopenic purpura (ITP) have similar problems. What common information can be provided to the parents of these children?

(832))   21. Identify a nursing diagnosis for a child with leukemia and nursing interventions that may be implemented.

(833)   22. For HIV infections:

The majority of children are infected: _____ .

The greatest physical threat is: _____ .

(833)   23. The mother of a child with HIV infection asks if the child should receive routine immunizations. The nurse responds by saying:

(834)   24. What are the priority nursing diagnoses for a child with juvenile rheumatoid arthritis?

Multiple Choice

(822)   25. A common sign or symptom of patent ductus arteriosus and septal defects is:
1. murmur.
2. chest pain.
3. hypotension.
4. headache.

(822)   26. The nurse recognizes that the majority of congenital heart defects are treated with:
1. diet.
2. exercise.
3. surgery.
4. medication.

(827)   27. Screenings are being conducted on children for blood disorders. The nurse is aware that the most prevalent blood disorder is:
1. hemophilia.
2. sickle cell anemia.
3. iron deficiency anemia.
4. idiopathic thrombocytopenic purpura.

(827)   28. The nurse instructs the parents of a child with iron deficiency anemia that iron absorption may be enhanced by:
1. giving the supplement with milk.
2. giving the supplement with citrus juice or fruits.
3. offering a chewable form once each day.
4. waiting until the child has a full stomach to administer.

(833)   29. HIV testing for a child who is less than 18 months of age is done with a:
1. Western blot test.
2. reticulocyte test.
3. polymerase chain reaction (PCR) test.
4. enzyme-linked immunosorbent assay (ELISA).

Student Name_____

RESPIRATORY

Objective

- Identify major alterations in respiratory function and specific nursing interventions for children with pneumonia.

(835)   30.   Respiratory distress syndrome (RDS) becomes apparent: _____.

(835)   31.   Treatment for RDS includes:

What are the general goals of medical treatment for children experiencing respiratory disorders?

(836)   32.   Identify the general nursing interventions that are implemented for children experiencing respiratory disorders.

(836)   33.   The largest percentage of pneumonia in children is caused by:

_____.

(837)   34.   The priority nursing intervention for parents of children with sudden infant death syndrome (SIDS) is:

(838)   35.   The new parent asks the nurse what the "Back to Sleep" campaign is all about. The nurse explains that this campaign is:

(838)   36. Acute pharyngitis is treated with: _____.

Diagnosis is based on: _____

Nursing measures include: _____

(839)   37. What is a classic sign of croup (laryngotracheobronchitis)?

(839)   38. Medical treatment for epiglottitis requires:

(841)   39. What is the pathophysiology involved in cystic fibrosis?

What is the medical management for this disorder?

(842)   40. One of the most frequent causes of bronchial asthma is:

_____.

(842)   41. For bronchial asthma, identify the following:

Signs/symptoms _____

Diagnostic tests _____

Medical treatment _____

Nursing interventions _____

Student Name _____

(844)   42.   The child is born with a cleft lip and palate. What are the primary problems for this child and the parents?

GASTROINTESTINAL

Objective

- Describe the clinical manifestations and medical management of children with gastrointestinal system dysfunctions.

(847)   43.   Identify the signs and symptoms of dehydration.

(847)   44.   Children with gastrointestinal disorders are prone to fluid and electrolyte imbalances. Identify the nursing assessments and interventions that should be implemented by the nurse for these children.

(848)   45.   Identify a nursing diagnosis for a child with diarrhea and/or dehydration.

(849)   46.   Identify how the diet may be modified for the following children who are experiencing constipation:

Newborn _____

Older infant _____

(850)   47.   The primary sign that is seen in children with hypertrophic pyloric stenosis is:

_____.

(852)   48.   The hallmark sign of intussusception is: _____.

(852)   49.   Treatment for intussusception includes:

(852)   50.   A neonate is suspected of having Hirschsprung's disease (megacolon) when:

_____.

(853)   51.   The usual surgical treatment for Hirschsprung's disease (megacolon) involves:

(852)   52.   What are general nursing measures that can be implemented for children experiencing gastrointestinal disorders?

(854)   53.   The nurse is aware that cultural practices related to hernias may include:

Multiple Choice

(847)   54.   For the child experiencing gastroenteritis with diarrhea, the nurse anticipates that treatment will include:
          1.   NPO.
          2.   oral rehydration.
          3.   no foods for 48 hours.
          4.   traditional BRAT diet.

Student Name _____

(854) 55. There are several different types of hernias that children may experience. The type of hernia that usually has spontaneous closure by the time the child is 2 years old is:
1. hiatal.
2. inguinal.
3. umbilical.
4. diaphragmatic.

(854) 56. The most severe type of hernia that is found within hours of delivery and requires immediate surgical repair is:
1. hiatal.
2. inguinal.
3. umbilical.
4. diaphragmatic.

GENITOURINARY

(855) 57. What are the signs and symptoms manifested by the child who has nephritic syndrome (nephrosis)?

(856) 58. Acute glomerulonephritis is most often the result of:

_____.

(856) 59. For acute glomerulonephritis, identify the following:

Signs/symptoms _____

Treatment _____

(857) 60. Wilms' tumor (nephroblastoma) is usually found by the parents when:

_____.

(857) 61. Treatment for Wilms' tumor includes:

Multiple Choice

(855)   62. The nurse is aware of the disease process and treatment for nephrosis. It is anticipated that treatment for the child will include:
1. prevention of infection.
2. increased sodium.
3. decreased protein.
4. diuretics.

(857)   63. The nurse expects that the treatment for a child with cryptorchidism will include:
1. circumcision.
2. fixation of the testes.
3. extension of the urethra.
4. bladder neck reconstruction.

ENDOCRINE

(858)   64. What are the signs and symptoms associated with acquired hypothyroidism?

(859)   65. The dietary needs of the child with hyperthyroidism include:

(859)   66. Most children with diabetes mellitus require: _____.

(860)   67. What information is necessary to include in a teaching plan for a newly diagnosed diabetic child and the parents?

Student Name_____

Multiple Choice

(859)   68. The nurse recognizes that hyperthyroidism is most common in which one of the following age groups?
1.   neonates
2.   toddlers
3.   preschoolers
4.   adolescents

MUSCULOSKELETAL

Objectives

- Demonstrate an understanding of the nursing interventions for the patient with congenital hip dysplasia.
- Describe five nursing interventions for a child in a corrective device or cast.

(860)   69. A hip dysplasia is suspected because of the presence of:

_____.

(862)   70. Identify the interventions that are important in the care of a cast or corrective device.

(861)   71. A child with Legg-Calvé-Perthes disease usually exhibits:

(863)   72. Scoliosis is: _____.

Scoliosis is most often seen in what age group? _____

Treatment usually includes:

(865)   73. The goals of treatment for a child with Duchenne's muscular dystrophy are:

Multiple Choice

(864)   74. For a child with talipes equinovarus, the nurse explains to the parents that treatment usually includes:
1. oxygen.
2. medication therapy.
3. skeletal traction.
4. cast applications.

NEUROLOGICAL

Objective

- List five clinical manifestations of meningitis.

(866)   75. For meningitis, identify the following:

Most common cause _____

Classic signs/symptoms _____

Diagnostic test _____

Medical treatment _____

Preventive measure _____

(867)   76. Hydrocephalus is:

(867)   77. For hydrocephalus, identify the following:

Appearance of the child _____

Medical treatment _____

Nursing interventions _____

(869)   78. What are the antenatal factors that may contribute to the development of cerebral palsy?

Student Name _____

(870)   79.   What are the nursing goals for a child with cerebral palsy?

(871)   80.   Identify whether the following interventions during a child's seizure are appropriate or require correction:

Keeping the side rails padded _____

Moving the child to the bed when the seizure begins _____

Loosened restrictive clothing _____

Turning the child's head to the side _____

Pushing a tongue blade between the teeth _____

Staying with the child throughout the seizure _____

(872)   81.   Nursing care for a child with a myelomeningocele includes:

(873)   82.   For lead poisoning, identify the following:

Sources of lead _____

Prevention _____

Screening _____

Parent guidelines to reduce lead levels _____

INTEGUMENTARY/COMMUNICABLE DISEASE

Objective

- Describe the clinical manifestations of common skin disorders in infants and children.

(875)   83. Identify some of the common areas for parent teaching for children with contact dermatitis, diaper rash, and eczema.

(877)   84. The skin disorder most commonly associated with adolescents is:

_____.

(878)   85. Identify a nursing diagnosis appropriate for a child with an integumentary disorder.

(879)   86. Identify actions that may be implemented to prevent traumatic injuries.

(880)   87. For a bacterial infection of the skin, identify an example of a nursing intervention.

(881)   88. The nurse is presenting information on parasitic infections to parents at a PTA meeting. What information should be included?

(882)   89. Which childhood communicable diseases may have cardiac complications?

Multiple Choice

(876)   90. A possible etiology associated with atopic dermatitis (eczema) is:
1. food allergy.
2. bacterial infection.
3. exposure to poison ivy.
4. increased sebaceous gland activity.

Student Name _____

SENSORY

Objective

- Identify methods of nursing assessment used to detect alterations in sensory organs.

(886) 91. For otitis media, identify the following:

Reason for common occurrence in children _____

Signs/symptoms _____

Nursing interventions _____

(886) 92. What behaviors usually indicate that a child may be having difficulty with vision?

(819) 93. Children experiencing health deviations and their parents may be referred to community agencies, organizations, and support groups. Identify at least three examples of available community resources.

CHAPTER 31

Care of the Child with a Mental or Cognitive Disorder

Answer Key: Textbook page references are provided as a guide for answering these questions. A complete answer key was provided for your instructor.

TERMS

Objective

- Define the key terms as listed.

    1.   Define the following terms:

(890)   Cognitive impairment _____

(893)   Failure to thrive _____

(890)   Intelligence quotient (IQ) _____

(896)   Somatization disorder _____

COGNITIVE DISORDERS

Objectives

- Identify six possible causes of cognitive impairment.
- Describe the clinical manifestations of Down syndrome.

(890)   2.   How are cognitive impairments classified?

(890)   3.   For cognitive impairments, identify the following:

          Possible etiology _____

          Clinical manifestations _____

Diagnostic testing _____

Nursing interventions _____

(891)   4.   In 95% of the instances, Down syndrome is the result of:

_____.

(891)   5.   Identify the clinical manifestations of Down syndrome:

(891)   6.   Medical care for the child with Down syndrome involves:

CHILD ABUSE

Objective

- State five physical and behavioral indicators that should arouse suspicion of child abuse.

(892)   7.   Identify the different types of neglect.

(892)   8.   What situational factors may contribute to child abuse?

(892)   9.   What is the role of the nurse regarding child abuse?

(893)   10.   Identify at least one behavioral and physical indicator for each of the following:

Physical neglect _____

Physical abuse _____

Sexual abuse _____

Emotional neglect and abuse _____

LEARNING/BEHAVIORAL DISORDERS

Objectives
- Demonstrate an understanding of the medical management and nursing interventions for the child with a learning disability.
- Describe four nursing interventions for the child with attention deficit hyperactivity disorder.

(894)   11.   The nurse believes that the child is experiencing school avoidance. What physiological and psychological assessment findings would lead to that belief?

(894)   12.   How can the nurse assist and support the parents if the child is experiencing school avoidance?

(894)   13.   For learning disabilities, identify the following:

Possible etiology _____

Clinical signs/symptoms _____

Medical/nursing intervention _____

(895)   14.   Management of an attention deficit hyperactivity disorder (ADHD) includes:

_____

(895)   15.   Nursing interventions for a child with ADHD include:

MENTAL DISORDERS

Objectives

- Identify six clinical manifestations of depression in children.
- Discuss three nursing interventions for the child who is suicidal.

(896)   16.   Describe depression and how it is diagnosed.

(896)   17.   In addition to medication, what treatment is provided for children who are depressed?

(896)   18.   Identify a nursing diagnosis for a child who is depressed.

(897)   19.   The nursing interventions for a child who is threatening or has attempted suicide include:

(897)   20.   The occurrence of recurrent abdominal pain (RAP) is mostly associated with:

Multiple Choice

(896)   21.   The nurse anticipates that the child who is depressed will receive which one of the following medications?
1. Prozac
2. Ritalin
3. Benadryl
4. Dexedrine

(897)   22.   The nurse is alert to careful screening for signs of suicidal thoughts or behaviors. The age group that is most prone to suicide is:
1. 5–7 years.
2. 8–11 years.
3. 12–14 years.
4. 15–19 years.

CHAPTER 32

Student Name _____

Health Promotion and Care of the Older Adult

Answer Key: Textbook page references are provided as a guide for answering these questions. A complete answer key was provided for your instructor.

TERMS

Objective

- Define the key terms as listed.

Match the terms in Column A with the appropriate definition or description in Column B.

Column A		Column B
(918)	1. _____ Akinesia	a. An abnormal curve in the upper spine
(918)	2. _____ Aphasia	b. Normal loss of hearing acuity, auditory threshold, and pitch
(918)	3. _____ Ataxia	c. Difficult, poorly articulated speech
(910)	4. _____ Claudication	d. Impaired ability to coordinate movement
(918)	5. _____ Dysarthria	e. Itching of the skin
(908)	6. _____ Dysphagia	f. Difficulty in swallowing
(911)	7. _____ Kyphosis	g. Cramping pain in the calves
(915)	8. _____ Presbycusis	h. Farsightedness resulting from a loss of elasticity of the lens
(914)	9. _____ Presbyopia	i. Abnormal state of motor and psychic hypoactivity
(905)	10. _____ Pruritus	j. Language function is absent or defective because of cerebral damage

OVERVIEW OF AGING

Objectives

- Discuss health and wellness in the aging population of the United States in relation to the aims of *Healthy People 2010*.
- Identify some of the common myths concerning the older adult.
- Describe biologic and psychosocial theories of aging.

(901)   11. It is estimated that by the year 2030, _____% of the population will be over 65 years of age.

(902)   12. Identify health promotion measures for the older adult.

(902)   13. There are many myths about older adults. Identify at least two of these myths.

(903)   14. The screenings that are recommended specifically for men over age 50 are:

(903)   15. The first major legislation for financial support of older adults was the:

_____. This legislation established the programs for:

_____.

(903)   16. The two most frequent indicators of elder abuse are:

_____.

(922)   17. The main goals of *Healthy People 2010* related to older adults are:

Student Name_____

Multiple Choice

(904)   18.   The theory of aging that presumes the personality of older adults remains the same and
                 behavior becomes more predictable is:
                 1.   activity theory.
                 2.   exchange theory.
                 3.   continuity theory.
                 4.   programmed aging.

PHYSIOLOGICAL CHANGES THAT OCCUR WITH AGING

Objectives

- Describe changes associated with aging for each of the body systems.
- Discuss methods of assessment used for each body system.
- Describe how older adults differ from younger individuals in their response to illness, medications, and hospitalization.
- Identify changes that occur with aging in intelligence, learning, and memory.

(905)   19.   Identify at least three changes in the integumentary system that occur with aging.

(905)   20.   Why is the older adult more susceptible to pressure ulcers?

(906)   21.   Identify at least three changes in the gastrointestinal system that occur with aging.

(907)   22.   Why is the older adult more susceptible to dehydration?

(907)   23.   The older adult may experience problems with oral hygiene, such as:

                 _____.

(909)   24.   Identify at least three changes in the urinary system that occur with aging.

(909)   25.   What are some of the common concerns related to urinary function for the older adult?

(910)   26.   Identify at least three changes in the cardiovascular system that occur with aging.

(911)   27.   Identify at least three changes in the respiratory system that occur with aging.

(911)   28.   What are some of the common concerns related to respiratory function for the older adult?

Student Name _____

(911)   29. Identify at least three changes in the musculoskeletal system that occur with aging.

(911)   30. What are the common concerns related to musculoskeletal function for the older adult?

(913)   31. Identify at least three changes in the endocrine system that occur with aging.

(913)   32. The majority of older adults experience _____ diabetes.

(913)   33. Identify at least three changes in the reproductive system that occur with aging.

(915)   34. Identify the changes that occur with the aging process in the following sensory areas:

Vision _____

Hearing_____

Taste/smell _____

(916)   35. An age-related change in the neurological function of the older adult is:

_____.

(917)   36. The goals for the patient with Alzheimer's disease are:

(918)   37. What is the difference between a transient ischemic attack (TIA) and a cerebrovascular accident (CVA)?

(919)   38. Metabolism of medications is decreased in the older adult as a result of:

Multiple Choice

(905)   39. A change that occurs in the integumentary system of the older adult is:
   1. decreased capillary fragility.
   2. increased hair pigmentation.
   3. increased sweat gland function.
   4. decreased vascularity of the dermis.

(906)   40. The recommended caloric intake for an average older adult is:
   1. 1000–1200 kcal/day.
   2. 1200–1500 kcal/day.
   3. 1800–2400 kcal/day.
   4. 3000 or more kcal/day.

(910)   41. Inadequate arterial circulation to the lower extremities of an older adult is usually evident with the presence of:
   1. edema.
   2. excessive warmth.
   3. bounding pulses.
   4. cramping of the calf muscles.

(920)   42. The effects of medications given to older adults may be altered as a result of:
   1. decreased adipose tissue.
   2. increased gastric secretions.
   3. increased total body water.
   4. increased sensitivity of brain receptors.

Student Name _____

PSYCHOSOCIAL CHANGES THAT OCCUR WITH AGING

Objectives
- Describe why finances and housing are major concerns for the older adult.
- Describe common psychosocial events that occur to the older adult.
- Describe ways to preserve dignity and to increase self-esteem of the older adult.

(917)   43. Social reminiscence involves:

(921)   44. Identify the concerns of the older adult related to the following:

Finances _____

Housing _____

(921)   45. Specify whether the following statements are true (T) or false (F).

Cognitive abilities decrease with old age. _____

Medication dosages for older adults may have to be reduced. _____

The majority of older adults reside in nursing homes. _____

A primary factor in the decreased sexual activity of the older adult is the lack of a sexual partner. _____

(921)   46. Losses experienced by the older adult may include:

(922)   47. A common response to loss in the older adult is: _____.

(923)   48. Evaluate whether the following communication is appropriate:

Calling the older woman "Grandma." _____

Addressing the older adult by the first name. _____

NURSING INTERVENTIONS

Objectives

- Identify nursing diagnoses appropriate to the older adult.
- Describe appropriate nursing interventions for common health concerns of the older adult.

(905)   49.   For the following systems, identify the nursing assessment of the older adult:

Integumentary _____

Cardiovascular _____

Respiratory _____

Gastrointestinal _____

Urinary _____

Musculoskeletal _____

Neurological _____

(908)   50.   Identify nursing interventions that may be implemented for the older adult who is experiencing constipation.

(910)   51.   What nursing interventions may be implemented for the patient with peripheral vascular disease?

(911)   52.   Identify a possible nursing diagnosis and interventions for an older adult experiencing respiratory changes.

Student Name_____

(912)　　53. What interventions should be implemented by the nurse to reduce the chance of falls for the older adult in an acute- or long-term care setting?

(913)　　54. How can the nurse promote an older adult's sexuality?

(914)　　55. Measures that should be used by the nurse to promote the patient's vision and hearing are:

(916)　　56. Reality orientation includes:

(919)　　57. Identify the nursing interventions for the older adult who is taking the following medications:

Antihypertensives _____

Diuretics _____

Opioids/narcotics _____

Multiple Choice

(909)   58. For the patient who is experiencing nocturia, the nurse intervenes by:
   1.   restraining the patient.
   2.   giving diuretics after 7:00 PM.
   3.   providing fluids at bedtime.
   4.   keeping the call bell within reach.

(905)   59. The older adult is experiencing pruritus. The nurse should:
   1.   apply water-based lotions.
   2.   use an antibacterial soap.
   3.   increase the frequency of bathing.
   4.   administer regular alcohol rubs.

(908)   60. For the older adult patient with dysphagia, the nurse should:
   1.   add thickeners to liquids.
   2.   feed the patient quickly to reduce fatigue.
   3.   place the patient in low Fowler's position for meals.
   4.   distract the patient by putting on music or the television.

(912)   61. The nurse anticipates that the patient who has osteoporosis will receive:
   1.   raloxifene.
   2.   Symmetrel.
   3.   Cognex.
   4.   Artane.

CHAPTER 33 Basic Concepts of Mental Health

Answer Key: Textbook page references are provided as a guide for answering these questions. A complete answer key was provided for your instructor.

TERMS

Objective

- Define the key terms as listed.

Match the terms in Column A with the appropriate definition or description in Column B.

	Column A		Column B
(930)	1. _____ Adaptation	a.	Pattern of behaviors that is conspicuous, threatening, and disruptive of relationships
(930)	2. _____ Affect	b.	Pertaining to body fluids or substances contained in them
(929)	3. _____ Anxiety	c.	Release of psychiatric patients to be treated in the community setting
(931)	4. _____ Defense mechanisms	d.	Relatively consistent attitudes and behaviors particular to an individual
(927)	5. _____ Deinstitutionalization	e.	Vague feeling of apprehension that results from a perceived threat to the self
(926)	6. _____ Humoral theory	f.	An individual's ability to adjust to changing life situations
(925)	7. _____ Mental health	g.	Unconscious, intrapsychic reactions that offer protection to the self
(925)	8. _____ Mental illness	h.	Ability to cope with and adjust to the recurrent stresses of everyday living
(928)	9. _____ Personality	i.	Nonspecific response of the body to any demand made on it
(929)	10. _____ Stress	j.	External manifestation of inner feeling or emotions

BASIC CONCEPTS

Objectives

- Describe the mental health continuum.
- Identify defining characteristics of persons who are mentally healthy and those who are mentally ill.
- Describe the parts of personality.
- Describe the factors that influence an individual's response to change.

(926)   11.   What is the emphasis of mental health nursing?

(926)   12.   In relation to treatment of mental illness, identify a major development or historical figure associated with the following time periods:

Greco-Roman period: _____

Dark ages: _____

Late 1700s–1800s: _____

1940s: _____

1970s: _____

(928)   13.   What is meant by a *mental health continuum*?

(928)   14.   Identify some general characteristics that are associated with mental illness.

(928)   15.   For the following theorists, identify the basic concepts of personality development:

Erikson _____

Freud _____

Student Name_____

(929)   16.   Identify the aspects of the self:

ALTERATIONS IN MENTAL HEALTH

Objectives

- Identify factors that contribute to the development of emotional problems or mental illness.
- Identify barriers to health adaptation.
- Identify sources of stress.
- Identify stages of illness behavior.
- Identify major components of a nursing assessment that focuses on mental health status.
- Identify basic nursing interventions for those experiencing illness or crisis.

(929)   17.   What are the types and effects of stressors on a person?

(929)   18.   Describe the difference in functioning from mild to high anxiety states.

(929)   19.   Identify the responses to the following:

Mild anxiety _____

Moderate anxiety _____

Severe anxiety _____

Panic _____

(930)   20.   Describe how motivation, frustration, conflicts, and coping abilities affect an individual.

(931)   21.   What are possible coping responses that may be used by individuals?

(932)   22.   Common behaviors seen in illness are:

(933)   23.   Identify examples of nursing diagnoses and patient outcomes that may be used in mental health nursing:

(933)   24.   What are the goals and steps in crisis intervention?

(933)   25.   What considerations should be made for the older adult in regard to mental health?

(934)   26.   Assessment of the patient's emotional state includes:

Multiple Choice

(931)   27.   The nurse is assessing an individual's use of defense mechanisms. One of the parents has had a bad day at work and comes home and shouts at the children. This is an example of:
1. projection.
2. displacement.
3. identification.
4. reaction formation.

(931)   28.   Regressive behavior is identified by the nurse when:
1. the victim of sexual abuse who laughs while telling about the incident.
2. an adolescent who participates in a lot of competitive sports.
3. an 80-year-old acts as if an incident of incontinence did not occur.
4. an 8-year-old begins sucking his thumb and wetting the bed when hospitalized for the first time.

CHAPTER 34

Care of the Patient with a Psychiatric Disorder

Answer Key: Textbook page references are provided as a guide for answering these questions. A complete answer key was provided for your instructor.

TERMS

Objective

- Define the key terms as listed.

Match the terms in Column A with the appropriate definition or description in Column B.

	Column A		Column B
(947)	1. _____ Compulsion	a.	Out of touch with reality, with severe personality deterioration
(944)	2. _____ Cyclothymic disorder	b.	False, fixed belief that cannot be corrected by feedback
(938)	3. _____ Delusion	c.	Mood disturbance characterized by feelings of sadness, despair, and lowered self-esteem
(943)	4. _____ Depression	d.	Pattern of repeated mood swings of hypomania and depression
(938)	5. _____ Hallucination	e.	Behavior performed in response to an obsessive thought
(944)	6. _____ Hypomanic episode	f.	Ineffective coping with stress that causes mild interpersonal disorganization
(948)	7. _____ Illusion	g.	Sensory experience without a stimulus trigger
(937)	8. _____ Neurosis	h.	Early phase of a bipolar episode when symptoms are not severe
(947)	9. _____ Obsession	i.	Irrational fear in which the individual tends to dwell on the object
(949)	10. _____ Paraphilia	j.	Uncommon and possibly illegal sexually gratifying activities
(947)	11. _____ Phobia	k.	False interpretation of extreme sensory stimulus, usually visual or auditory
(937)	12. _____ Psychosis	l.	Thought that is recurrent, intrusive, and senseless

MENTAL DISORDERS

Objectives

- List the five axes of DSM-IV-TR used to examine and treat mental illnesses.
- Identify and describe the major mental disorders.
- List five warning signs of suicide.

(937)   13.   What is the difference between neurosis and psychosis?

(937)   14.   What is the purpose of the *Diagnostic and Statistical Manual of Psychiatric Disorders, IV-TR?*

(937)   15.   For the DSM-IV-TR, identify the axis:

Major psychiatric disorders: Axis _____

Psychiatric and environmental disorders: Axis _____

General medical conditions relevant to mental disorders: Axis _____

(938)   16.   For organic mental disorders, what is the difference between delirium and dementia?

(939)   17.   Identify and briefly describe the major mental disorders.

Student Name_____

(942) 18. Match the terms for behaviors seen in schizophrenia in Column A with the appropriate descriptions of the behaviors in Column B.

Column A   **Column B**

(942)   _____ Disordered   a.   Inability to experience happiness or joy
                        thinking   b.   Reduced content of speech
                                          c.   Inability to interpret information being
(942)   _____ Apathy   received
                                          d.   Lack of energy
(942)   _____ Alogia   e.   Lack of nonverbal expression of emotions

(942)   _____ Flat affect

(942)   _____ Anhedonia

(943) 19. Identify the following types of delusions that are exhibited:

"The man on the radio is telling me to buy that car."_____

"That other patient put the idea in my head." _____

"They are listening to my conversations through the intercom."

_____

(943) 20. What are the subtypes of schizophrenia?

(944) 21. Identify the warning signs of suicide.

(945) 22. What are the signs and symptoms of a panic attack?

(948)   23.   Identify the different types of personality disorders:

(949)   24.   Behavior that indicates a persistent desire to be the opposite sex is termed:

_____.

TREATMENT

Objectives

- Identify basic interventions for patients experiencing various mental health problems.
- Describe the general care and treatment methods for patients experiencing mental health problems.
- Name two alternative medicines used for mental disorders.

(939)   25.   Identify the treatment and nursing interventions for the major mental disorders.

(939)   26.   What are some of the commonalities in nursing interventions for patients with mental disorders?

(941)   27.   For a patient with a mood or anxiety disorder, the nurse can decrease stimuli by:

Student Name _____

(945)   28.   What are specific treatments for patients who are depressed?

(945)   29.   Identify precautions that should be taken for patients who are suicidal:

(951)   30.   Identify whether the following statements are appropriate when preparing a patient for electroconvulsive therapy (ECT):

Pain will be experienced. _____

Confusion will decrease after a few hours. _____

Grand mal seizures are experienced. _____

Most patients are kept in the hospital for 2–3 days after. _____

(945)   31.   What medications are typically used for depression?

(946)   32.   Identify possible patient outcomes for an individual who is experiencing depression:

(948)   33.   The patient in the clinic escaped the World Trade Center disaster on September 11, 2001.

The nurse is alert to the possible development of: _____.

Signs and symptoms of this disorder are:

(949) 34. The patient has come to the physician's office with nausea, vomiting, and stomach pain. The patient tells the nurse that she just got a new job with a lot of responsibilities, many people to supervise, and two projects that are due within the month. The nurse suspects that this patient may be experiencing:

(949) 35. The nurse who is working with patients with sexual disorders should first:

(950) 36. While completing an admission history, the patient asks the nurse not to tell anyone that he wants to end his life. The nurse should respond by:

(950) 37. What are the different types of psychotherapy?

(953) 38. For the following, identify examples of medications, side effects, and nursing actions:

Antipsychotics _____

Antidepressants _____

(955) 39. Identify examples of alternative therapies and their uses:

Multiple Choice

(940) 40. Communication with a patient who is in the manic phase of a bipolar affective disorder should:
1. reinforce assertive behaviors.
2. provide focus and consistency.
3. offer verbal reminders of the day and date.
4. encourage lengthy expression of thoughts and feelings.

Student Name _____

(941)   41. The nurse anticipates that the patient with an obsessive-compulsive disorder will receive:
1. lithium.
2. Haldol.
3. Thorazine.
4. Anafranil.

(940)   42. The nurse is aware that a patient who is receiving lithium therapy needs to have an adequate intake of:
1. calcium.
2. sodium.
3. magnesium.
4. potassium.

(939)   43. A patient tells you that he is hearing voices right now that are telling him not to eat. The nurse's best response is:
1. "What did the voices tell you not to eat?"
2. "Did the voices say that you couldn't even eat snacks?"
3. "I don't think that the voices would tell you not to eat anything."
4. "I don't hear any voices. Tell me what you are experiencing now."

CHAPTER 35

Care of the Patient with an Addictive Personality

Answer Key: Textbook page references are provided as a guide for answering these questions. A complete answer key was provided for your instructor.

TERMS

Objective

- Define the key terms as listed.

Match the terms in Column A with the appropriate definition or description in Column B.

		Column A		Column B
(959)	1.	_____ Addiction	a.	Drug that alters perception and thinking
(971)	2.	_____ Amotivational cannabis syndrome	b.	Decreased goal-directed activities, abrupt mood swings, and apathy
			c.	Drug dependence and substance abuse
(970)	3.	_____ Bruxism	d.	Removal of the poisonous effects of a substance from a patient
(963)	4.	_____ Detoxification	e.	Grinding of the teeth
(961)	5.	_____ Gateway drug	f.	Increase in the amount and frequency of drug use to achieve the same effect
(969)	6.	_____ Hallucinogen	g.	Agent that increases the rate of body activity
(971)	7.	_____ Huffing	h.	Substance that is used first that leads to abuse of other substances
(960)	8.	_____ Psychoactive drug	i.	Inhaling solvents that have been put on a cloth or into a bag
(969)	9.	_____ Stimulant	j.	Substance that makes the user feel good
(960)	10.	_____ Tolerance		

ADDICTION

Objectives

- Name two traits attributed to an addictive personality.
- Describe the three stages of dependence.
- Describe one legal effort that has decreased the incidence of substance abuse.

(959)   11. What are the four elements of addiction?

(959)   12. An amazing statistic is that _____% of children who begin drinking at or before the age of 14 develop alcoholism.

_____% of all motor vehicle accident deaths and fatal injuries are associated with alcohol.

(960)   13. In relation to drugs, how has federal law influenced the health care provider?

(960)   14. Identify examples of behaviors seen in the early, middle, and late stages of dependence.

(963)   15. When completing a nursing assessment, identify examples of the subjective and objective data that may be indicative of substance abuse.

(963)   16. What diagnostic tests may be used to determine the possibility of substance abuse?

Student Name_____

(964)   17.   Identify examples of possible nursing diagnoses and outcomes for addicted patients who have physical and emotional needs:

(964)   18.   What support groups are available for individuals who are seeking to stop their addictive behavior?

(965)   19.   The goal of treatment centers is: _____.

ALCOHOLISM

Objectives

- Describe three disorders associated with alcoholism.
- Explain the two phases of recovery: detoxification and rehabilitation.

(961)   20.   What are some of the possible contributing factors to alcoholism?

(961)   21.   Alcohol is classified as a: _____.

(961)   22.   One of the reasons that binge drinking by college students is such a hazard is because rapid, large-quantity consumption of alcohol can lead to:

_____.

(961)   23.   Identify the electrolyte and nutritional imbalances that may occur with alcoholism and the reason they occur.

(962)   24. What complications or problems are associated with fetal alcohol syndrome?

(962)   25. For the following disorders associated with alcoholism, identify the signs and symptoms and when they usually begin to be seen:

Alcohol withdrawal syndrome:

Delirium tremens:

Korsakoff's psychosis and Wernicke's encephalopathy:

(962)   26. Identify the effects that alcohol has on the following body systems:

Gastrointestinal _____

Hepatic _____

Cardiovascular _____

Respiratory _____

Musculoskeletal _____

(964)   27. For the phases of recovery, identify the nursing interventions that should be implemented:

Acute/detoxification _____

Rehabilitation _____

Multiple Choice

(962)   28. A patient has a blood alcohol level of 475 mg/dl (0.475%). The nurse expects that this patient will exhibit:
1. stupor or coma.
2. stumbling and blurred vision.
3. clumsiness and emotional changes.
4. mild sedation with pleasant, relaxed attitude.

Student Name_____

DRUG ABUSE

Objective

- Identify six types of drugs of abuse.

(967)   29.   Substance abuse affects what part of the brain?

         This may alter the person's _____.

(967)   30.   Identify the signs and symptoms of central nervous system (CNS) depressants:

(967)   31.   Identify at least six commonly used drugs:

(968)   32.   What drugs have been associated with "date rape"?

(968)   33.   The most widely abused opioid is: _____.

(968)   34.   For opioids, identify the signs and symptoms of an overdose and withdrawal.

(968)   35.   What is the use of methadone?

         What drug is having better effects than methadone?

(968)   36.   Identify the different types of stimulants:

(968)   37.   What are the signs and symptoms of stimulant use?

(969)   38.   Medications that are used to decrease the craving for cocaine are:

(969)   39.   The nurse is assessing a patient who is suspected of chronic cocaine abuse. The nurse will expect to find:

(969)   40.   What are the complications of amphetamine use?

Student Name _____

(969)   41.   A patient has been abusing a hallucinogen. What serious problems may this patient develop?

(970)   42.   What signs and symptoms may be seen with the use of ecstasy (MDMA)?

                  What makes this drug so dangerous for abuse?

(970)   43.   Cannabis is also known as: _____.

                  Identify possible effects of its use:

(971)   44.   Identify examples of gateway drugs:

(971)   45.   What are some of the common effects of inhalant use?

Multiple Choice

(968)   46. A coworker states that he has had too much caffeine and wants to eliminate it from his diet. He should be advised to drink:
1. coffee.
2. cola drinks.
3. orange juice.
4. hot chocolate.

(968)   47. The patient is quitting smoking cigarettes. The withdrawal from nicotine may result in the patient having:
1. lethargy.
2. improved concentration.
3. decreased heart rate.
4. decreased appetite.

(971)   48. The nurse is working with patients who have abused the following substances. Which one is NOT expected to cause withdrawal signs and symptoms?
1. cannabis
2. CNS stimulants
3. CNS depressants
4. hallucinogens

IMPAIRED NURSE

Objective

-   Describe steps taken to help the chemically impaired nurse.

(973)   49. The chemically impaired nurse may exhibit the same signs and symptoms of abuse as any other individual who is addicted. What are the specific role-related signs or behaviors that may be seen by coworkers?

(973)   50. Identify the assistance that is available for the chemically impaired nurse:

(973)   51. What is the Healthcare Integrity and Protection Data Bank (HIPDB)?

CHAPTER 36 Home Health Nursing

Answer Key: Textbook page references are provided as a guide for answering these questions. A complete answer key was provided for your instructor.

TERMS

Objective

- Define the key terms as listed.

    1.   Define the following:

(978)   Medicare _____

(978)   Medicaid _____

OVERVIEW/TRENDS

Objectives

- List at least three types of home health agencies.
- Discuss new developments that are occurring in home health care.

(977)   2.   Identify the historical developments in home health care associated with the following dates:

    1600s _____

    1796 _____

    1893 _____

    1909 _____

    1935 _____

    1965 _____

    1983 _____

(978)   3.   What special considerations are made by the nurse in regard to the older adult and home care?

(979)   4.   For the following types of home health agencies, identify an example and who they are governed by:

Voluntary _____

Official _____

Proprietary _____

(978)   5.   What are some of the regulations that must be followed by home health agencies?

(980)   6.   Identify at least two of the changes that are occurring in home health care:

(987)   7.   What factors have increased the need for home health care?

SERVICES

Objectives

- Describe how home health care differs from community and public health care services.
- List at least four services that may be provided by home health care.
- Describe two major ways home care differs from hospital care.
- Define skilled nursing services.
- Describe the role of the LPN/LVN in the delivery of skilled nursing care.

Student Name_____

- Relate the nursing process to home health care practice.
- Relate seven steps to breaking through cultural barriers to communication.

(980)   8.   Identify the types of services that are provided by home health agencies:

(981)   9.   What is meant by *skilled nursing care*?

(981)   10.   The service goals of home health nursing are:

(981)   11.   The role of the LPN/LVN in home health care is:

(983)   12.   Where do home health care referrals usually come from?

(983)   13. What are the steps in the home health care process once the patient is referred?

(983)   14. Identify what is included in the admission of a patient to the home health care agency.

(983)   15. What type of documentation is used in home health care and what methods may be used to complete it?

(984)   16. The major principles of total quality management or quality improvement are:

(986)   17. Identify the steps that may be taken to break through the cultural barriers to communication.

Student Name _____

Multiple Choice

(982)   18. The home health nurse will refer the patient who requires promotion of independence
with the use of a self-help device to the:
1.   social worker.
2.   physical therapist.
3.   home health aide.
4.   occupational therapist.

REIMBURSEMENT

Objectives

- Summarize governmental financing for home health nursing.
- List two sources of reimbursement for home care services.

(976)   19. Identify the effect that federal financing has had on home health care since 1997.

(981)   20. Medicare and Medicaid require that the plan of treatment is:

_____.

(982)   21. What are the Medicare requirements for the following services?

Physical therapy _____

Speech therapy _____

Home health aide _____

(984)   22. Identify the different types of reimbursement sources for home health care and provide an
example of eligibility criteria for one of the sources.

CHAPTER 37

Student Name _____

Long-Term Care

Answer Key: Textbook page references are provided as a guide for answering these questions. A complete answer key was provided for your instructor.

TERMS

Objective

- Define the key terms as listed.

Match the terms in Column A with the appropriate definition or description in Column B.

Column A	Column B
(992) 1. _____ Activities of daily living	a. Landmark legislation affecting long-term care facilities
(993) 2. _____ Adult day care	b. Setting that provides subacute care
(994) 3. _____ Assisted living	c. Terminal care agency or setting
(992) 4. _____ Hospice	d. Community-based programs designed to meet needs that require less than 24-hour care
(994) 5. _____ Instrumental activities of daily living	e. Measure of the optimum energy or force that allows a person to cope successfully with a wide range of challenges
(996) 6. _____ Omnibus Budget Reconciliation Act (OBRA)	f. Hygiene, dressing, grooming, toileting, eating, and ambulating
(990) 7. _____ Quality of life	g. Institutional setting that provides a less expensive alternative to hospital-based care
(994) 8. _____ Residential care	h. Settings that offer living facilities
(995) 9. _____ Subacute unit	i. More complex tasks such as shopping and using the telephone
(995) 10. _____ Skilled nursing facility	j. Residential care setting where adult patient rents a small apartment or bedroom area

REGULATIONS AND REIMBURSEMENT

Objectives

- Discuss federal and state regulations related to long-term care.
- Identify the sources of reimbursement for long-term care services.

(996)   11.   What did the Omnibus Budget Reconciliation Act of 1987 do for long-term care?

(997)   12.   What did OBRA do for the LPN/LVN in long-term care?

(997)   13.   Identify the legal and ethical issues related to long-term care:

(997)   14.   What sources of reimbursement are available for long-term care facilities?

PATIENTS AND SERVICES

Objectives

- Describe settings of long-term care services.
- Identify patients of long-term care services.
- Define chronic and acute health services.
- Describe goals of long-term care health services.
- Describe long-term care nursing services.
- Describe services available from each type of agency: home health agency, hospice agency, adult day care, assisted living facility, continuing care community, long-term care facility.

Student Name _____

(991) 15. What are some of the cultural and ethnic considerations for long-term care?

(991) 16. Identify the different settings for long-term care and provide an example of each type.

(992) 17. For the patient who has a terminal disease, the appropriate referral is to a:

(993) 18. The patient requires stimulation and supervision while her daughter is at work. What type of setting is recommended?

(994) 19. Assisted living offers what types of services for its residents?

(994) 20. How does a continuing care retirement community differ from assisted living?

(995)   21. Identify the advantages or benefits associated with subacute care:

(995)   22. What is the profile of the patient who requires long-term care in an institutional setting?

(996)   23. Identify how the administration of medications differs in long-term care facilities:

(997)   24. What is the purpose of a Resident Assessment Instrument (RAI) and what is involved in the assessment?

(998)   25. How does documentation in a long-term care facility differ from that in a hospital setting?

Student Name_____

(998)   26. Identify a nursing diagnosis for a resident in a long-term care facility who has safety needs.

(999)   27. Identify the usual time frame for the following nursing activities in a long-term care facility:

Making rounds to monitor residents _____

Reviewing the plan of care _____

Charting for a resident who has no change in status _____

CHAPTER 38

Rehabilitation Nursing

Answer Key: Textbook page references are provided as a guide for answering these questions. A complete answer key was provided for your instructor.

TERMS

Objective

- Define the key terms as listed.

    1. Define the following terms:

(1003)   Interdisciplinary rehabilitation team _____

(1003)   Multidisciplinary rehabilitation team _____

(1003)   Transdisciplinary rehabilitation team _____

REHABILITATION NURSING

Objectives

- Define the philosophy of rehabilitation nursing.
- Describe the interdisciplinary rehabilitation team concept and the function of each team member.
- Discuss specialized practice characteristics of the rehabilitation nurse.

(1001)   2.   Identify the philosophy of rehabilitation nursing:

(1002)   3.   What are the different needs for rehabilitation?

(1002)   4.   Identify a general goal of rehabilitation:

(1003)   5.   Who are the members of the rehabilitation team and what are their roles?

(1004)   6.   Describe the role of the rehabilitation nurse:

(1004)   7.   For the comprehensive rehabilitation plan:

The plan is started _____

The plan is reevaluated _____

The plan is developed based upon _____

Multiple Choice

(1002)   8.   Two patients are admitted to a rehabilitation hospital. Both have the same medical condition, but one patient is not able to manage, physically or emotionally, the adaptation required. This patient is best described as having a:
1.   disability.
2.   handicap.
3.   chronic illness.
4.   functional limitation.

DISABLING DISORDERS

Objectives

- Discuss two major disabling conditions.
- Provide nursing diagnoses, goals, interventions, and evaluation/outcome criteria for two major disabling conditions.

Student Name_____

(1006)   9.   What are two of the major disabling conditions?

(1006)   10. Define the following terms:

Quadriplegia_____

Paraplegia _____

Paresis _____

(1007)   11. For the following problems associated with spinal cord injuries, describe what happens, the signs and symptoms that are seen, and the nursing interventions:

Postural hypotension _____

Autonomic dysreflexia _____

Heterotopic ossification _____

Deep vein thrombosis_____

(1010)   12. What are the two types of head injuries?

(1009)   13. Identify the characteristic rehabilitation needs of patients who have suffered traumatic brain injuries:

(1010)   14. In the rehabilitative assessment of a patient following a traumatic brain injury (TBI), the nurse may expect to find:

(1009)   15.   For patients having a spinal cord injury or a traumatic brain injury, identify possible nursing diagnoses and outcomes:

Multiple Choice

(1008)   16.   The patient experienced a spinal cord injury at the T6–T9 level. The nurse anticipates that the patient should be able to:
1.   assist with ADLs.
2.   ambulate independently.
3.   drive with hand controls.
4.   control bowel and bladder function.

(1008)   17.   The construction worker sustained an injury to C7 after a fall at a work site. The nurse anticipates that this patient will be:
1.   nonambulatory.
2.   ADL independent.
3.   independent in bladder care.
4.   returning to prior job responsibilities.

(1010)   18.   The emergency squad brought in the patient following an accident at home. One of the squad members tells the nurse that the patient, according to the spouse, was unconscious for $1\frac{1}{2}$ hours. This head injury is described as:
1.   mild.
2.   moderate.
3.   severe.
4.   catastrophic.

ISSUES IN REHABILITATION

Objectives

- Discuss the importance of returning home and preparing for community reentry.
- Recognize the importance and significance of family-centered care in rehabilitation.
- Recognize the uniqueness of pediatric and gerontological rehabilitation nursing.

(1001)   19.   What are some of the current issues in rehabilitation?

Student Name _____

(1002)   20.   Identify the cornerstones of rehabilitation:

(1005)   21.   Identify the key elements of family-centered care:

(1006)   22.   How are pediatric and gerontological rehabilitation different from adult rehabilitation?

CHAPTER 39

Hospice Care

Answer Key: Textbook page references are provided as a guide for answering these questions. A complete answer key was provided for your instructor.

TERMS

Objective

- Define the key terms as listed.

Match the terms in Column A with the appropriate definition or description in Column B.

Column A

(1018)   1. _____ Adjuvant

(1021)   2. _____ Cachexia

(1015)   3. _____ Holistic

(1014)   4. _____ Palliative care

(1015)   5. _____ Primary caregiver

(1016)   6. _____ Respite

(1013)   7. _____ Terminal illness

(1018)   8. _____ Titrate

Column B

a.   Period of relief from responsibilities of caring for a patient

b.   Not curative in nature but designed to relieve pain and distress

c.   One who assumes ongoing responsibility for health maintenance and therapy for the illness

d.   Pertaining to the total person

e.   Advanced stage of disease with no known cure and poor prognosis

f.   Malnutrition marked by weakness and emaciation

g.   Additional drug or treatment that is added to assist in the action of the primary pain treatment

h.   Slowly increasing the amount of a drug to find the therapeutic dose

PHILOSOPHY AND ORGANIZATION

Objectives

- Discuss the philosophy of hospice care.
- Differentiate between palliative care and curative care.
- Name the members of the interdisciplinary team and explain their roles.
- Discuss the role of hospice in families' bereavement period.

(1013)   9.   What was the origin of the concept of hospice care?

(1014)   10.   The focus and the goals of hospice care are:

(1015)   11.   Identify the professionals in the core interdisciplinary hospice team and their roles:

(1022)   12.   What is the purpose of the bereavement team?

HOSPICE PATIENTS AND COMMON SYMPTOMS

Objectives

- Discuss four criteria for admission to hospice care.
- List three common symptoms related to a terminal illness.
- Discuss the usefulness of pain assessments and when assessments should be completed.
- Develop a care plan with patient goals related to these symptoms.

(1014)   13.   The usual criteria for admission of a patient to hospice are:

Student Name_____

(1019)   14.   What is included in a pain assessment?

(1019)   15.   In addition to assessment, what are the other nursing responsibilities for management of a hospice patient's pain?

(1018)   16.   For pain relief or reduction, identify the types of medications that may be used for the following:

Mild to moderate pain _____

Severe pain _____

Long-lasting results _____

(1019)   17.   In addition to pharmacologic therapy, the nurse recognizes that the following measures may also be implemented to relieve or reduce pain:

(1019)   18.   For the other common symptoms of a terminal illness, identify the nursing interventions:

Nausea and vomiting _____

Constipation_____

Anorexia and malnutrition _____

Dyspnea or air hunger _____

Weight loss, dehydration, and weakness_____

(1022)   19.   An appropriate response for the hospice nurse in determining the patient's spiritual needs is to:

(1022)   20.   Identify signs and symptoms of approaching death and the appropriate nursing interventions:

ISSUES

Objective

- Discuss two ethical issues in hospice care.

(1023)   21.   Identify ethical and legal issues that are associated with hospice care.

CHAPTER 40

Professional Roles and Leadership

Answer Key: Textbook page references are provided as a guide for answering these questions. A complete answer key was provided for your instructor.

TERMS

Objective

- Define the key terms as listed.

    1.   Define the following terms:

(1030)   Advancement _____

(1042)   Burnout _____

(1035)   Endorsement _____

(1036)   Nurse Practice Act _____

(1045)   Transcribe _____

CAREER PLANNING

Objectives

- Discuss the three methods of applying for a job.
- Describe what can be expected from an interview for a new job.
- Discuss career opportunities for the LPN/LVN.
- List the advantages of membership in professional organizations.
- Discuss telephone manners in professionalism.
- Identify strategies for burnout prevention.

(1026)   2.   Identify the steps in career planning for the LPN/LVN:

(1028)   3.   What are the guidelines for preparing a letter of application for a position?

(1028)   4.   The purpose and components of a good resume are:

(1029)   5.   How can you prepare for a successful interview?

(1029)   6.   What specific communication techniques should be employed for a successful interview?

(1030)   7.   Identify if the interviewer is allowed to ask you about the following:

Job-related criminal convictions _____

Financial or credit status _____

Marital status _____

Age _____

Educational background _____

Reason for leaving your prior employment _____

(1029)   8.   What is usually included in an employment contract?

Student Name_____

(1031)   9.   Identify the organizations that represent LPN/LVNs and their major functions:

(1033)   10.   What is the purpose of continuing education and what types are usually offered?

(1033)   11.   The LPN/LVN who wants to continue his/her formal professional education should

investigate: _____.

(1033)   12.   What types of certification are available to the LPN/LVN?

(1045)   13.   Appropriate telephone communication regarding physician's orders involves:

(1036)   14.   Identify possible career opportunities for the LPN/LVN:

(1038)   15.   An LPN/LVN who wishes to have flexible working hours and conditions should investigate:

(1039)   16.   Identify the areas that the following LPNs/LVNs are involved in:

An auto manufacturing plant _____

Working with the terminally ill _____

Working in the community _____

(1043)   17.   Identify the signs and symptoms of burnout and strategies that may be implemented to prevent this problem:

BOARD OF NURSING

Objectives

- Describe the Nurse Practice Act.
- Identify three important functions of a state board of nursing.
- List four reasons a state board of nursing could revoke a nursing license.
- Discuss the computerized adaptive testing (CAT) for the National Council Licensure Examination (NCLEX) for the LPN/LVN candidate.

(1034)   18.   For the NCLEX-PN examination, identify the following:

Minimum number of questions: _____

Maximum number of questions: _____

Maximum time allowed: _____

Goal of CAT testing: _____

Average time to receive results: _____

Approval to take the test given by: _____

(1036)   19.   Identify the role and functions of a state board of nursing:

Student Name _____

(1036)   20.   The state board of nursing may revoke a nurse's license for the following reasons:

LEADERSHIP

Objectives

- Explain the structure and role of the charge nurse.
- Discuss the guidelines for being an effective leader.
- Discuss styles of leadership that may be used by nurses.
- Discuss the duties of a nurse team leader.

(1039)   21.   Identify the type of leadership style that is being described:

Leader relinquishes all control and delegates responsibility to the group:

People-centered approach that allows employees to have more control and participation in decision-making:

Leader retains all authority and responsibility having one-way communication with the group:

Takes into account the style of the leader and the characteristics of the group:

(1041)   22.   What is the usual role of a team leader?

(1041)   23.   Identify the guidelines for effective leadership:

(1042)   24.   Principles of time management include:

(1042) 25. The LPN is working with another staff member who has not done what she was supposed to do for the patient. This is not the first time that this has occurred and the LPN is becoming angry. What should this LPN do?

Multiple Choice

(1040) 26. There has been an earthquake in the area and the disaster victims are being brought into the emergency room. In this situation, the type of leadership that is the most effective for the nurse manager is:
1. democratic.
2. autocratic.
3. situational.
4. laissez-faire.

LEGAL ISSUES

Objectives

- Discuss confidentiality.
- List the three types of physician's orders and discuss the legal aspects of each.
- List three ways you can ensure accuracy when transcribing physician's orders.
- List the pertinent data necessary to compile an effective end-of-shift report.

(1044) 27. What precautions should be taken by the nurse when transcribing physician's orders?

(1044) 28. For the following, identify if the action is appropriate:

The nurse is unsure of the order that is written, but believes that it is appropriate and transcribes it to the medication administration record. _____

The nurse administers a preoperative treatment to a patient the afternoon following the surgery. _____

A discontinued medication is crossed out with a highlighting marker. _____

(1046) 29. For a change-of-shift report, identify the following:

Purpose _____

Methods _____

Information to include _____

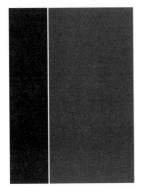

Skills Performance Checklists

These checklists were developed to assist in evaluating the competence of students in performing the nursing interventions presented in the text *Foundations of Nursing*. The checklists are perforated for easy removal and reference. Students can be evaluated with a "Satisfactory" or "Unsatisfactory" performance rating by putting a check in the appropriate column for each step. Specific instruction or feedback can be provided in the "Comments" column. All the checklists have been streamlined to include **only** the critical steps needed to satisfactorily master the skill. They are **not** intended to replace the text, which describes and illustrates each nursing skill in detail.

Student Name _____ Date _____ Instructor's Name _____

PERFORMANCE CHECKLIST 9-1

CARE OF THE BODY AFTER DEATH

		S	U	Comments
1.	Assemble appropriate equipment	❑	❑	_____
2.	Wash hands	❑	❑	_____
3.	Don clean gloves	❑	❑	_____
4.	Close patient's eyes and mouth as necessary	❑	❑	_____
5.	Remove all tubings and other devices from around patient's body unless contraindicated	❑	❑	_____
6.	Place patient in supine position (do not place one hand on top of the other)	❑	❑	_____
7.	Elevate the head			
8.	Replace soiled dressings with clean ones	❑	❑	_____
9.	Bathe patient as necessary (place absorbent pad under buttocks)	❑	❑	_____
10.	Brush or comb hair	❑	❑	_____
11.	Apply clean gown	❑	❑	_____
12.	Care for valuables (jewelry) and personal belongings	❑	❑	_____
13.	Allow family to view body and remain in room if family wishes	❑	❑	_____
14.	After the family has left the room, attach special label if patient had a contagious disease	❑	❑	_____
15.	Close door to room	❑	❑	_____
16.	Await arrival of ambulance or transfer to morgue; some agencies use a shroud to enclose the body before transfer to morgue	❑	❑	_____
17.	If shroud is to be used, enclose body into shroud at this time	❑	❑	_____

		S	U	Comments
18.	Document procedure and disposition of patient's body as well as belongings and valuables	❏	❏	_____

Student Name _____ Date _____ Instructor's Name _____

PERFORMANCE CHECKLIST 10-1

ADMITTING A PATIENT

	S	U	Comments
1. Wash hands	❑	❑	_____
2. Prepare the room			
a. Care items in place	❑	❑	_____
b. Bed at proper height and opened	❑	❑	_____
c. Light on	❑	❑	_____
3. Greet the patient and family; introduce self, roommate; project interest and concern	❑	❑	_____
4. Identify patient	❑	❑	_____
5. Assess immediate needs	❑	❑	_____
6. Orient the patient to the unit: lounge and nurses' station	❑	❑	_____
7. Orient the patient to the room: call light, bed controls, telephone, and television	❑	❑	_____
8. Explain hospital routines	❑	❑	_____
9. Provide privacy, assist to undress as necessary	❑	❑	_____
10. Properly care for valuables, clothing, and medications	❑	❑	_____
11. Obtain the patient's health history, and do the initial nursing assessment correctly	❑	❑	_____
12. Provide for safety: bed in low position, side rails up, call light within easy reach	❑	❑	_____
13. Begin care as ordered by the physician	❑	❑	_____
14. Invite the family back into the room if they left earlier	❑	❑	_____
15. Wash hands	❑	❑	_____

	S	U	Comments
16. Record the information correctly	❏	❏	_____
17. Provide the patient and the family time for privacy	❏	❏	_____
18. Do patient teaching	❏	❏	_____

PERFORMANCE CHECKLIST 10-2

TRANSFERRING A PATIENT

		S	U	Comments
1.	Wash hands	❑	❑	_____
2.	Check physician's order	❑	❑	_____
3.	Inform the patient and family of transfer	❑	❑	_____
4.	Notify receiving unit of patient transfer	❑	❑	_____
5.	Gather the patient's belongings and necessary care items	❑	❑	_____
6.	Assist in transferring the patient	❑	❑	_____
7.	Properly introduce patient and family to new unit: nurses and roommate	❑	❑	_____
8.	Provide a brief summary of medical diagnoses, treatment care plan, and medication; review medical orders with nurse assuming care. If transfer is to another facility, complete an interagency transfer form correctly	❑	❑	_____
9.	Explain equipment, policies, and procedures that are different on the new unit	❑	❑	_____
10.	Wash hands	❑	❑	_____
11.	Record condition of patient and means of transfer	❑	❑	_____
12.	Notify other hospital departments as necessary	❑	❑	_____
13.	For an interagency transfer, dress the patient appropriately	❑	❑	_____
14.	If patient is a child, adjust procedure appropriately	❑	❑	_____
15.	Do patient teaching	❑	❑	_____

PERFORMANCE CHECKLIST 10-3

DISCHARGING A PATIENT

		S	U	Comments
1.	Wash hands	❏	❏	_____
2.	Verify discharge order	❏	❏	_____
3.	Arrange for patient or family to visit business office as necessary	❏	❏	_____
4.	If no discharge order has been written, have patient sign appropriate AMA form	❏	❏	_____
5.	Notify the family or person who will be transporting the patient home	❏	❏	_____
6.	Make certain patient and family understand instructions	❏	❏	_____
7.	Gather equipment, supplies, and prescriptions that the patient is to take home	❏	❏	_____
8.	Check to see that business office has given a release	❏	❏	_____
9.	Assist the patient in dressing and packing items to go home	❏	❏	_____
10.	Check clothing and valuables list made on admission	❏	❏	_____
11.	Transfer the patient and belongings via wheelchair to the vehicle; assist patient into the vehicle if needed	❏	❏	_____
12.	Wash hands	❏	❏	_____
13.	Chart discharge procedure	❏	❏	_____
14.	If patient is a child, adjust procedure as appropriate	❏	❏	_____

PERFORMANCE CHECKLIST 11-1

MEASURING BODY TEMPERATURE

		S	U	Comments
1.	Wash hands	❏	❏	_____
2.	Assess for signs and symptoms of temperature alterations and for factors that influence body temperature	❏	❏	_____
3.	Introduce self to patient	❏	❏	_____
4.	Identify patient	❏	❏	_____
5.	Explain procedure to patient	❏	❏	_____
6.	Prepare for procedure			
a.	Assemble the appropriate thermometer and other necessary supplies	❏	❏	_____
b.	Provide privacy	❏	❏	_____
c.	Determine whether patient has consumed hot or cold beverage or food or has been smoking	❏	❏	_____
7.	Obtaining an oral temperature: electronic thermometer			
a.	Wash hands and don gloves	❏	❏	_____
b.	Remove thermometer pack from charging unit; remove probe from storage well of recording unit	❏	❏	_____
c.	Insert probe snugly into probe cover—red probe for rectal readings, blue probe for oral and axillary readings	❏	❏	_____
d.	Inspect digital display	❏	❏	_____
e.	Request that patient open mouth and gently insert probe correctly; request that patient hold thermometer in place with lips closed	❏	❏	_____
f.	Wait for audible signal	❏	❏	_____

		S	U	Comments
g.	Remove probe from patient's mouth and remove probe cover and dispose correctly	❏	❏	_____
h.	Provide for patient comfort	❏	❏	_____
i.	Read and write down reading	❏	❏	_____
j.	Return thermometer to storage unit	❏	❏	_____
k.	Wash hands	❏	❏	_____
l.	Document findings	❏	❏	_____

8. Obtaining rectal temperature: electronic thermometer

		S	U	Comments
a.	Wash hands	❏	❏	_____
b.	Assist patient to the Sims' position	❏	❏	_____
c.	Don gloves	❏	❏	_____
d.	Remove thermometer pack from charging unit; make certain correct rectal probe is attached to the unit and slide disposable plastic cover over thermometer probe	❏	❏	_____
e.	Lubricate thermometer probe	❏	❏	_____
f.	Gently spread buttocks and insert thermometer probe appropriately; hold on to thermometer throughout procedure	❏	❏	_____
g.	Hold electronic probe until audible signal occurs	❏	❏	_____
h.	Read temperature on digital display; remove probe from rectum and dispose of plastic cover appropriately	❏	❏	_____
i.	Return probe to storage unit and later return the unit to its charging device	❏	❏	_____
j.	Clean anal area of lubricant and possible feces; remove and dispose of gloves and wash hands	❏	❏	_____
k.	Assist patient to a position of comfort	❏	❏	_____
l.	Write down reading	❏	❏	_____
m.	Document findings	❏	❏	_____

Student Name _____ Date _____ Instructor's Name _____

		S	**U**	**Comments**

9. Obtaining axillary temperature: electronic thermometer

    a. Wash hands ❑ ❑ _____

    b. Assist patient to supine or sitting position ❑ ❑ _____

    c. Expose axilla; make certain the area is clean and dry ❑ ❑ _____

    d. Prepare electronic thermometer ❑ ❑ _____

    e. Insert probe into the correct area and position body part correctly ❑ ❑ _____

    f. Hold electronic probe until audible signal occurs and read digital display ❑ ❑ _____

    g. Remove probe from patient's axilla; remove probe cover and dispose correctly ❑ ❑ _____

    h. Return electronic probe to storage well ❑ ❑ _____

    i. Assist patient to regown and position for comfort ❑ ❑ _____

    j. Wash hands ❑ ❑ _____

    k. Return thermometer to charger base ❑ ❑ _____

    l. Write down reading ❑ ❑ _____

    m. Document findings ❑ ❑ _____

10. Obtaining tympanic temperature: electronic thermometer

    a. Wash hands ❑ ❑ _____

    b. Assist patient to an appropriate position ❑ ❑ _____

    c. Remove hand-held thermometer unit from charging base ❑ ❑ _____

    d. Slide disposable plastic speculum cover over otoscope-like tip ❑ ❑ _____

    e. Follow manufacturer's instructions for tympanic probe positioning ❑ ❑ _____

			S	**U**	**Comments**
	(1)	Gently tug ear pinna up and back for an adult; down and back for a child	❏	❏	_____
	(2)	Move thermometer gently in a figure-eight fashion	❏	❏	_____
	(3)	Fit ear probe snugly into canal	❏	❏	_____
	(4)	Point toward the nurse, following manufacturer's positioning recommendations	❏	❏	_____
f.		Depress scan button on hand-held unit and read assessment	❏	❏	_____
g.		Carefully remove sensor from ear and push release button to eject plastic speculum cover discarding in proper receptacle	❏	❏	_____
h.		Return hand-held unit to charging base	❏	❏	_____
i.		Assist patient to a comfortable position	❏	❏	_____
j.		Wash hands	❏	❏	_____
k.		Write down reading	❏	❏	_____
l.		Document findings	❏	❏	_____
11.		Postprocedure for measuring body temperature			
a.		Compare temperature findings with baseline and normal temperature range for patient's age group	❏	❏	_____
b.		If temperature is abnormal, repeat procedure; if indicated, choose alternate site or instrument for second reading	❏	❏	_____
c.		Record temperature on vital sign flow sheet/graphic sheet/nurse's notes correctly and report abnormal findings to nurse in charge or physician	❏	❏	_____
d.		Do patient teaching	❏	❏	_____

Student Name _____ Date _____ Instructor's Name _____

PERFORMANCE CHECKLIST 11-2

OBTAINING A PULSE RATE

		S	U	Comments
1.	Wash hands	❑	❑	_____
2.	Introduce self	❑	❑	_____
3.	Identify patient	❑	❑	_____
4.	Explain procedure	❑	❑	_____
5.	Prepare for procedure			
a.	Assemble all necessary supplies	❑	❑	_____
b.	Provide privacy	❑	❑	_____
6.	Implement procedure			
a.	Count pulse for 60 seconds	❑	❑	_____
b.	Palpate pulse			
(1)	Radial pulse correctly	❑	❑	_____
(2)	Ulnar pulse correctly	❑	❑	_____
(3)	Brachial pulse correctly	❑	❑	_____
(4)	Femoral pulse correctly	❑	❑	_____
(5)	Popliteal pulse correctly	❑	❑	_____
(6)	Dorsalis pedis pulse correctly	❑	❑	_____
(7)	Posterior tibial pulse correctly	❑	❑	_____
c.	Determine strength of pulse	❑	❑	_____
7.	Write down rate	❑	❑	_____
8.	Wash hands	❑	❑	_____
9.	Document rate correctly	❑	❑	_____
10.	Follow up by reporting any abnormal pulse rates	❑	❑	_____
11.	Do patient teaching	❑	❑	_____

PERFORMANCE CHECKLIST 11-3

OBTAINING AN APICAL PULSE RATE

		S	U	Comments
1.	Wash hands	❏	❏	_____
2.	Introduce self	❏	❏	_____
3.	Identify patient	❏	❏	_____
4.	Explain procedure	❏	❏	_____
5.	Prepare for procedure			
	a. Assemble all necessary supplies	❏	❏	_____
	b. Provide privacy	❏	❏	_____
6.	Implement procedure			
	a. Clean stethoscope as recommended	❏	❏	_____
	b. Position patient and expose patient's chest as necessary	❏	❏	_____
	c. Place stethoscope against patient's chest in correct position	❏	❏	_____
	d. Count pulse rate correctly	❏	❏	_____
	e. Provide comfort	❏	❏	_____
7.	Write down pulse rate	❏	❏	_____
8.	Wash hands	❏	❏	_____
9.	Document rate correctly	❏	❏	_____
10.	Report any abnormal pulse rates	❏	❏	_____
11.	Do patient teaching	❏	❏	_____

PERFORMANCE CHECKLIST 11-4

OBTAINING A RESPIRATORY RATE

		S	U	Comments
1.	Wash hands	❏	❏	_____
2.	Introduce self	❏	❏	_____
3.	Identify patient	❏	❏	_____
4.	Explain procedure	❏	❏	_____
5.	Prepare for procedure			
a.	Assemble all necessary supplies	❏	❏	_____
b.	Provide privacy	❏	❏	_____
c.	If patient has been active, wait the recommended time	❏	❏	_____
d.	Position patient comfortably	❏	❏	_____
6.	Implement procedure			
a.	Place fingertip as if to obtain a radial pulse	❏	❏	_____
b.	Observe and count respiratory rate correctly	❏	❏	_____
c.	Provide comfort	❏	❏	_____
7.	Write down rate	❏	❏	_____
8.	Wash hands	❏	❏	_____
9.	Document rate correctly	❏	❏	_____
10.	Report abnormal rates	❏	❏	_____
11.	Do patient teaching	❏	❏	_____

PERFORMANCE CHECKLIST 11-5

OBTAINING A BLOOD PRESSURE READING

		S	U	Comments
1.	Wash hands	❏	❏	_____
2.	Introduce self	❏	❏	_____
3.	Identify patient	❏	❏	_____
4.	Explain procedure	❏	❏	_____
5.	Determine if patient has ingested caffeine or has been smoking and wait the suggested length of time	❏	❏	_____
6.	Prepare for procedure			
	a. Assemble all necessary supplies	❏	❏	_____
	b. Determine correct cuff size	❏	❏	_____
	c. Position patient correctly	❏	❏	_____
	d. Provide privacy	❏	❏	_____
	e. Determine site for blood pressure measurement	❏	❏	_____
7.	Implement procedure			
	a. Apply cuff correctly	❏	❏	_____
	b. Palpate radial artery	❏	❏	_____
	c. Inflate cuff, determine approximate systolic pressure	❏	❏	_____
	d. Deflate the cuff correctly	❏	❏	_____
	e. Palpate the brachial artery and place the stethoscope bell/diaphragm correctly	❏	❏	_____
	f. Correctly reinflate cuff	❏	❏	_____
	g. Correctly deflate cuff	❏	❏	_____

		S	U	Comments
h.	Accurately determine blood pressure reading while listening to Korotkoff sounds	❏	❏	_____
i.	Completely deflate and remove the cuff	❏	❏	_____
j.	Provide comfort	❏	❏	_____
8.	Write down rate	❏	❏	_____
9.	Wash hands	❏	❏	_____
10.	Document reading correctly	❏	❏	_____
11.	Report abnormal readings	❏	❏	_____
12.	Do patient teaching	❏	❏	_____

Student Name _____ Date _____ Instructor's Name _____

PERFORMANCE CHECKLIST 11-6

MEASURING HEIGHT AND WEIGHT

		S	U	Comments
1.	Wash hands	❏	❏	_____
2.	Introduce self	❏	❏	_____
3.	Identify patient	❏	❏	_____
4.	Explain procedure	❏	❏	_____
5.	Prepare for procedure			
	a. Assemble supplies	❏	❏	_____
	b. Provide privacy	❏	❏	_____
6.	Implement procedure			
	a. Balance scales at zero and place paper towel for patient to stand on	❏	❏	_____
	b. Assist patient onto scales correctly	❏	❏	_____
	c. Measure height correctly	❏	❏	_____
	d. Measure weight correctly	❏	❏	_____
	e. Assist patient off scales correctly	❏	❏	_____
	f. Provide comfort	❏	❏	_____
7.	Write down measurements	❏	❏	_____
8.	Wash hands	❏	❏	_____
9.	Document measurements	❏	❏	_____
10.	Report measurements if required	❏	❏	_____
11.	Do patient teaching	❏	❏	_____

PERFORMANCE CHECKLIST 12-1

PERFORMING A 2-MINUTE HANDWASHING

		S	U	Comments
1.	Inspect hands	❑	❑	_____
2.	Determine contaminant of hands	❑	❑	_____
3.	Assess areas around the hands that are contaminated or clean	❑	❑	_____
4.	Explain to the patient the importance of handwashing	❑	❑	_____
5.	Remove jewelry (except plain wedding band) and push watch and long sleeves above wrists	❑	❑	_____
6.	Adjust the water to appropriate temperature and force	❑	❑	_____
7.	Wet hands and wrists, keeping hands lower than elbows	❑	❑	_____
8.	Lather hands	❑	❑	_____
9.	Wash hands appropriately	❑	❑	_____
10.	Wash 1 minute thoroughly, rinse thoroughly, re-lather and wash another minute using a continuous amount of friction	❑	❑	_____
11.	Rinse wrists and hands completely	❑	❑	_____
12.	Clean fingernails correctly with nail file and orangewood stick	❑	❑	_____
13.	Dry hands thoroughly	❑	❑	_____
14.	Turn off faucets appropriately	❑	❑	_____
15.	Use hand lotion	❑	❑	_____
16.	Inspect hands and nails for cleanliness	❑	❑	_____
17.	Do patient teaching	❑	❑	_____

PERFORMANCE CHECKLIST 12-2

Gloving

	S	U	Comments

Donning Gloves

		S	U	Comments
1.	Obtain gloves from dispenser	❏	❏	_____
2.	Inspect gloves for perforation	❏	❏	_____
3.	Don gloves as recommended	❏	❏	_____
4.	Change gloves after direct handling of infectious material such as wound drainage	❏	❏	_____
5.	Do not touch side rails, tables, or bed stands with contaminated gloves	❏	❏	_____

Removing Gloves

		S	U	Comments
6.	Remove first glove appropriately	❏	❏	_____
7.	Remove second glove appropriately	❏	❏	_____
8.	Wash hands	❏	❏	_____
9.	Do patient teaching	❏	❏	_____

PERFORMANCE CHECKLIST 12-3

GOWNING FOR ISOLATION

		S	U	Comments
1.	Remove watch and push up long sleeves	❏	❏	_____
2.	Place watch on a paper towel or see-through baggie before taking vital signs	❏	❏	_____
3.	Wash hands	❏	❏	_____
4.	Obtain, don, and secure gown properly	❏	❏	_____
5.	When finished with patient care, remove gown appropriately	❏	❏	_____
6.	Discard soiled gown appropriately	❏	❏	_____
7.	Wash hands	❏	❏	_____
8.	Record use of gown	❏	❏	_____
9.	Do patient teaching	❏	❏	_____

PERFORMANCE CHECKLIST 12-4

DONNING A MASK

		S	U	Comments
1.	Obtain a mask	❏	❏	_____
2.	Don and secure mask correctly	❏	❏	_____
3.	Wear mask for recommended period of time	❏	❏	_____
4.	Make certain patient feels comfortable and accepted by nurse	❏	❏	_____
5.	Remove mask correctly	❏	❏	_____
6.	Dispose of soiled mask appropriately	❏	❏	_____
7.	Wash hands thoroughly	❏	❏	_____
8.	Record use of mask	❏	❏	_____
9.	Do patient teaching	❏	❏	_____

Student Name _____ Date _____ Instructor's Name _____

PERFORMANCE CHECKLIST 12-5
DOUBLE BAGGING

		S	U	Comments
1.	Don gown, mask, and gloves before entering patient's room	❏	❏	_____
2.	Assemble all contaminated disposable articles in isolation bag	❏	❏	_____
3.	Summon second health care worker who remains outside the room	❏	❏	_____
4.	Second person hold double bag with top edge of bag covering hands	❏	❏	_____
5.	First person drops contaminated bag in double bag without touching	❏	❏	_____
6.	Secure and label bags appropriately	❏	❏	_____
7.	First person places new bags in holders	❏	❏	_____
8.	Remove gloves, gown, and mask without contamination	❏	❏	_____
9.	Wash hands thoroughly	❏	❏	_____
10.	Record double-bagging procedure	❏	❏	_____
11.	Document patient's response to isolation	❏	❏	_____
12.	Do patient teaching	❏	❏	_____

PERFORMANCE CHECKLIST 12-6

ISOLATION TECHNIQUE

		S	**U**	**Comments**
1.	Determine causative microorganism	❑	❑	_____
2.	Recognize mode of transmission and how microorganism exits the body	❑	❑	_____
3.	Follow agency policy for specific type of isolation used	❑	❑	_____
4.	Provide an environment with adequate equipment and supplies:			
	a. Private room or isolation with anteroom	❑	❑	_____
	b. Sign stating isolation category	❑	❑	_____
	c. Adequate handwashing facilities	❑	❑	_____
	d. Special containers for trash, soiled linen, and sharp instruments such as needles	❑	❑	_____
5.	Plan time to explain isolation technique to patient, family, and visitors	❑	❑	_____
6.	Post card on door of patient's room or wall outside room stating the protective measures in use for patient care	❑	❑	_____
7.	Supply the room with designated lined containers for soiled linens and for trash	❑	❑	_____
8.	Assess vital signs, administer medication, administer hygiene, and collect specimens all in the appropriate manner	❑	❑	_____
9.	Report changes in the patient's health status	❑	❑	_____
10.	Record assessments and performance of protective asepsis	❑	❑	_____
11.	Determine patient's level of understanding and do patient teaching	❑	❑	_____

PERFORMANCE CHECKLIST 12-7

PREPARING A STERILE FIELD

		S	U	Comments
1.	Prepare sterile field just before planned procedure	❏	❏	_____
2.	Select clean work surface above waist level	❏	❏	_____
3.	Assemble necessary equipment			
	a. Sterile drape	❏	❏	_____
	b. Assorted sterile supplies	❏	❏	_____
4.	Determine package sterility	❏	❏	_____
5.	Wash hands thoroughly	❏	❏	_____
6.	Place pack containing sterile drape on work surface and open without contamination	❏	❏	_____
7.	With fingertips of one hand, pick up folded top edge of sterile drape	❏	❏	_____
8.	Gently lift drape up from its outer cover and let it unfold by itself without touching any object; discard outer cover with your other hand	❏	❏	_____
9.	With other hand, grasp adjacent corner of drape and hold it straight up and away from your body	❏	❏	_____
10.	Holding drape, first position the bottom half over intended work surface	❏	❏	_____
11.	Allow top half of drape to be placed over work surface last	❏	❏	_____
12.	Perform procedure using sterile technique	❏	❏	_____

PERFORMANCE CHECKLIST 12-8

PERFORMING OPEN STERILE GLOVING

		S	U	Comments
1.	Obtain proper-sized sterile gloves	❏	❏	_____
2.	Perform thorough handwashing	❏	❏	_____
3.	Remove outer glove package wrapper by carefully separating and peeling apart sides	❏	❏	_____
4.	Grasp inner package and lay it on clean, flat surface just above waist level; open package, keeping gloves on wrapper's inside surface	❏	❏	_____
5.	Identify right and left glove; glove dominant hand first	❏	❏	_____
6.	With thumb and first two fingers of nondominant hand, grasp edge of glove cuff for dominant hand; touch only glove's inside surface	❏	❏	_____
7.	Carefully pull glove over dominant hand, leaving cuff and being sure cuff does not roll up wrist	❏	❏	_____
8.	With gloved dominant hand, slip fingers underneath second glove's cuff	❏	❏	_____
9.	Carefully pull second glove over nondominant hand	❏	❏	_____
10.	After second glove is on, interlock hands together	❏	❏	_____

Glove Disposal

		S	U	Comments
11.	Grasp outside of one cuff with other gloved hand	❏	❏	_____
12.	Pull glove off, turning it inside out; discard in receptacle	❏	❏	_____
13.	Take fingers of bare hand and tuck inside remaining glove cuff; peel glove off inside out; discard in receptacle	❏	❏	_____

PERFORMANCE CHECKLIST 12-9

PREPARING FOR DISINFECTION AND STERILIZATION

		S	U	Comments
1.	Prepare equipment and assemble supplies			
	a. Disinfectant to use for cleansing	❏	❏	_____
	b. Method of sterilization	❏	❏	_____
	c. Gloves	❏	❏	_____
	d. Running water	❏	❏	_____
	e. Scrub brush	❏	❏	_____
	f. Cloth wrapper	❏	❏	_____
2.	Don gloves	❏	❏	_____
3.	Rinse article under cool running water	❏	❏	_____
4.	Wash article with detergent	❏	❏	_____
5.	Use scrub brush to remove material in grooves	❏	❏	_____
6.	Dry article thoroughly	❏	❏	_____
7.	Prepare article for sterilization by wrapping it	❏	❏	_____
8.	Clean work area and put in order	❏	❏	_____
9.	Do patient teaching	❏	❏	_____

PERFORMANCE CHECKLIST 13-1

APPLYING SAFETY REMINDER DEVICES

		S	U	Comments
1.	Review medical record for orders	❏	❏	_____
2.	Wash hands	❏	❏	_____
3.	Introduce self	❏	❏	_____
4.	Identify patient	❏	❏	_____
5.	Explain procedure	❏	❏	_____
6.	Prepare for procedure by providing privacy and assembling necessary supplies	❏	❏	_____
7.	Assess patient for need of SRD	❏	❏	_____
8.	Apply appropriate type of SRD			
	a. Wrist or ankle (extremity) SRD			
	(1) If using Kerlix gauze, make a clove hitch correctly	❏	❏	_____
	(2) Pad the extremity appropriately	❏	❏	_____
	(3) Slip the wrist(s) or ankle(s) through loops directly over the padding; if using a commercially made SRD, wrap the padded portion of the device around affected extremity, thread tie through slit in SRD, and fasten to second tie with a secure knot correctly	❏	❏	_____
	(4) Secure ends of ties properly	❏	❏	_____
	(5) Leave as much slack as possible	❏	❏	_____
	(6) Palpate pulses below the SRD	❏	❏	_____
	b. Elbow SRD			
	(1) Place SRD over the elbow(s)	❏	❏	_____

		S	U	Comments
(2)	Wrap SRD snugly, tying the SRD at the top. For small infants, tie or pin SRDs to their shirts	❏	❏	_____
c.	Vest			
(1)	Apply device over the patient's gown	❏	❏	_____
(2)	Put vest on patient with V-shaped opening in the front	❏	❏	_____
(3)	Pull tie at end of vest flap across the chest, and slip tie through slip on opposite side of vest	❏	❏	_____
(4)	Wrap the other end of the flap across patient and secure the straps properly	❏	❏	_____
(5)	Allow enough space between the vest and the patient appropriately	❏	❏	_____
d.	Gait or safety reminder belts			
(1)	Apply belt over patient's gown	❏	❏	_____
(2)	If patient is ambulating, place belt around the patient's waist	❏	❏	_____
(3)	If the belt does not have a buckle, fasten in slip knot	❏	❏	_____

9. A quick-release knot rather than a regular knot should be used to secure the safety reminder devices to bed frame ❏ ❏ _____

10. Secure SRDs so that the patient cannot unfasten them ❏ ❏ _____

11. Apply SRD with gentleness and compassion ❏ ❏ _____

12. Wash hands ❏ ❏ _____

13. Document procedure completely and accurately ❏ ❏ _____

14. Follow-up

    a. Monitor for skin impairment ❏ ❏ _____

		S	U	Comments
b.	With the use of extremity SRD, assess extremity distal to SRD at least every 2 hours	❏	❏	_____
	(1) Remove SRD on one extremity at a time at least every 2 hours for 5 minutes	❏	❏	_____
c.	Monitor position of SRD, circulation, and skin condition	❏	❏	_____
d.	With the use of vest SRD, monitor respiratory status	❏	❏	_____
e.	SRD should be removed at least every 2 hours; patient should NOT be left unattended during this time	❏	❏	_____
f.	Massage skin beneath SRD; lotion or powder may be applied	❏	❏	_____
g.	SRD should be changed when soiled or wet	❏	❏	_____
h.	Check frequently for tangled ties or pressure points from knots; adjust SRD device(s) as needed	❏	❏	_____
i.	Monitor and document physical and mental status, circulation, and need for SRD; SRDs should be removed when they are no longer needed	❏	❏	_____
j.	If SRD use is necessary because of changes in the patient's condition, document the changes and efforts to calm or safeguard the patient without SRD use	❏	❏	_____
k.	Assess for any related problems	❏	❏	_____

15. Evaluation

		S	U	Comments
a.	The SRD is adequate and appropriate for the individual patient's condition	❏	❏	_____
b.	SRDs are correctly applied	❏	❏	_____
c.	Tied knots are easily released	❏	❏	_____

	S	U	Comments
d. Related problems, such as to the skin or the musculoskeletal system, are identified	❏	❏	_____
16. Do patient teaching	❏	❏	_____

PERFORMANCE CHECKLIST 14-1

POSITIONING PATIENTS

		S	U	Comments
1.	Assess patient's body alignment	❏	❏	_____
2.	Assemble equipment and supplies	❏	❏	_____
3.	Request assistance as needed	❏	❏	_____
4.	Introduce self	❏	❏	_____
5.	Identify patient	❏	❏	_____
6.	Explain procedure	❏	❏	_____
7.	Wash hands	❏	❏	_____
8.	Prepare patient			
	a. Close doors	❏	❏	_____
	b. Raise level of bed	❏	❏	_____
	c. Remove pillows	❏	❏	_____
	d. Position bed flat or as patient is able to tolerate	❏	❏	_____
9.	Position patient			
	a. Dorsal supine position			
	(1) Place patient on back with head flat	❏	❏	_____
	(2) Place small rolled towel under lumbar spine	❏	❏	_____
	(3) Place pillow under upper shoulders, neck, and head	❏	❏	_____
	(4) Place trochanter roll or sandbag along lateral surface of thighs	❏	❏	_____
	(5) Place small pillow or roll under back of ankle	❏	❏	_____

	S	U	Comments
(6) Support feet in dorsiflexion	❑	❑	_____
(7) Place pillow under forearms	❑	❑	_____
(8) Place hand rolls in patient's hands	❑	❑	_____
b. Dorsal recumbent			
(1) Lower head of bed	❑	❑	_____
(2) Move patient and mattress to head of bed	❑	❑	_____
(3) Turn patient onto back	❑	❑	_____
(4) Assist patient to raise legs, bend knees, and allow legs to relax	❑	❑	_____
(5) Replace pillow	❑	❑	_____
c. Fowler's			
(1) Move patient and mattress to head of bed	❑	❑	_____
(2) Raise head of bed to 45–60 degrees	❑	❑	_____
(3) Replace pillow	❑	❑	_____
(4) Use foot board	❑	❑	_____
(5) Use pillows to support arms and hands if needed	❑	❑	_____
(6) Place small pillow or roll under ankles	❑	❑	_____
d. Semi-Fowler's			
(1) Move patient and mattress to head of bed and remove pillow	❑	❑	_____
(2) Raise head of bed to 30 degrees	❑	❑	_____
(3) Replace pillow	❑	❑	_____
e. Orthopneic			
(1) Elevate head of bed to 90 degrees	❑	❑	_____

		S	U	Comments
(2)	Place pillow between patient's back and mattress	❏	❏	_____
(3)	Place pillow on overbed table and assist patient to lean over, placing head on pillow	❏	❏	_____

f. Sims'

		S	U	Comments
(1)	Place patient in supine position	❏	❏	_____
(2)	Place patient in left lateral position, lying partially on the abdomen	❏	❏	_____
(3)	Draw right knee and thigh up near abdomen	❏	❏	_____
(4)	Place patient's left arm along back	❏	❏	_____
(5)	Bring right arm up, flex elbow, and support with pillow	❏	❏	_____
(6)	Allow patient to lean forward to rest on chest	❏	❏	_____

g. Prone

		S	U	Comments
(1)	Assist patient onto abdomen with face to one side	❏	❏	_____
(2)	Flex arms toward the head	❏	❏	_____
(3)	Position pillows for comfort	❏	❏	_____

h. Knee-chest (genupectoral)

		S	U	Comments
(1)	Turn patient onto abdomen	❏	❏	_____
(2)	Assist patient to kneeling position; arms and head should rest on pillow while upper chest rests on bed	❏	❏	_____

i. Lithotomy

		S	U	Comments
(1)	Request patient to slide buttocks to the edge at end of examining table	❏	❏	_____
(2)	Lift both legs, have patient bend knees, and place feet in stirrups	❏	❏	_____

	S	U	Comments
(3) Drape patient appropriately	❏	❏	_____
(4) May need a small lumbar pillow	❏	❏	_____
j. Trendelenburg's			
(1) Place patient's head lower than body with body and legs elevated and on an incline (foot of bed may be elevated on blocks)	❏	❏	_____
10. Reassess patient for:			
a. Proper body alignment	❏	❏	_____
b. Comfort	❏	❏	_____
c. Skin integrity	❏	❏	_____
d. Respiratory difficulty	❏	❏	_____
e. Tolerance of position	❏	❏	_____
f. Reposition every 2 hours	❏	❏	_____
11. Wash hands	❏	❏	_____
12. Record appropriate alignment and position of patient	❏	❏	_____

PERFORMANCE CHECKLIST 14-2

PERFORMING RANGE-OF-MOTION EXERCISES

	S	U	Comments
1. Refer to medical record, care plan, or Kardex for special interventions	❏	❏	_____
2. Wash hands	❏	❏	_____
3. Introduce self	❏	❏	_____
4. Identify patient	❏	❏	_____
5. Explain procedure	❏	❏	_____
6. Prepare for procedure by providing privacy and assembling necessary supplies	❏	❏	_____
7. Assist patient in putting each joint through full ROM, appropriately supporting the body part being exercised	❏	❏	_____
a. Neck—Place palm of each hand against side of patient's face, or place one hand under patient's head and one hand on patient's chin			
(1) Bring head forward until chin touches sternum	❏	❏	_____
(2) Return head to straight position and have patient look straight ahead	❏	❏	_____
(3) Bend head backward with chin positioned toward ceiling	❏	❏	_____
(4) Return head to extension	❏	❏	_____
(5) Bend head laterally with ear toward shoulder, first toward right ear then left ear	❏	❏	_____
b. Shoulder—Cup one hand beneath elbow, and grasp wrist with other hand			
(1) Bring arm away from body	❏	❏	_____

		S	U	Comments
(2)	Return arm toward side of body	❏	❏	_____
(3)	Abduct the arm; continue movement until patient's hand is toward head of bed	❏	❏	_____
(4)	Abduct arm to shoulder level	❏	❏	_____

c. Elbow—Support patient's arm by grasping center of forearm with one hand and just above elbow with other hand

		S	U	Comments
(1)	Bend lower arm toward biceps	❏	❏	_____
(2)	Straighten lower arm	❏	❏	_____
(3)	Hold patient's hand as if to shake hands, and turn palm upward	❏	❏	_____
(4)	Continue holding patient's hand, and turn palm of hand downward	❏	❏	_____

d. Wrist—Hold wrist joint with one hand, and hold palm of patient's hand with other hand

		S	U	Comments
(1)	Bend wrist toward lower arm with fingers pointing downward	❏	❏	_____
(2)	Return wrist to a straight position	❏	❏	_____
(3)	Bend wrist with fingers pointing upward toward ceiling	❏	❏	_____
(4)	Extend wrist, and bend it laterally toward ulna side	❏	❏	_____

e. Fingers—Place palm and fingers of one hand directly against back of patient's hand and fingers

		S	U	Comments
(1)	Curve fingers with nurse's fingers to resemble a fist	❏	❏	_____
(2)	Straighten all fingers	❏	❏	_____
(3)	Using thumb and index finger of one hand, spread fingers apart by moving each one away from nearest finger	❏	❏	_____

	S	**U**	**Comments**

(4) Return fingers together until touching each other ❏ ❏ _____

f. Thumb—Hold patient's thumb with nurse's thumb and index finger

    (1) Manipulate thumb across the palm of hand to touch tip of each finger to tip of patient's thumb ❏ ❏ _____

    (2) Move thumb away from index finger return thumb toward index finger ❏ ❏ _____

    (3) Move thumb joint forward and backward ❏ ❏ _____

g. Hip—Support under knee joint with one hand, and grasp ankle joint with other hand

    (1) Raise leg with knee straight; return leg to bed in straight position ❏ ❏ _____

    (2) Raise leg and bend knee toward chest to flex to 110–120 degrees; straighten knee and return to bed ❏ ❏ _____

    (3) Move leg out away from midline ❏ ❏ _____

    (4) Bring leg back toward other leg ❏ ❏ _____

    (5) Position legs straight and roll leg outward, toes pointing outward ❏ ❏ _____

    (6) Position legs straight and roll leg inward, toes pointing toward each other ❏ ❏ _____

h. Knee—Support under knee joint with one hand, and grasp ankle joint with the other hand ❏ ❏ _____

    (1) Bend knee with calf touching thigh ❏ ❏ _____

    (2) Straighten knee ❏ ❏ _____

    (3) Extend knee beyond the normal point of extension ❏ ❏ _____

		S	U	Comments
(4)	Rotate knee and lower leg toward midline	❑	❑	_____
i.	Ankle—Grasp heel in palm of one hand, touching inner aspect of the forearm to the sole of the foot; support top of foot just above ankle with other hand			
(1)	Gently press against the sole of the foot with inner arm, toes pointing upward	❑	❑	_____
(2)	Press on top of foot to point toes downward	❑	❑	_____
(3)	Turn foot away from midline	❑	❑	_____
(4)	Turn foot inward	❑	❑	_____
j.	Toes—Place fingers over toes; support bottom of foot with hand and bottom of toes with other hand			
(1)	Curl toes downward toward bottom of foot	❑	❑	_____
(2)	Raise toes to point upward	❑	❑	_____
(3)	Spread toes apart	❑	❑	_____
(4)	Return toes toward each other	❑	❑	_____
8.	Position patient for comfort	❑	❑	_____
9.	Adjust bed linens	❑	❑	_____
10.	Remove and dispose of gloves and wash hands	❑	❑	_____
11.	Documentation			
a.	Report and record abnormal findings	❑	❑	_____
b.	Report and record normal findings	❑	❑	_____

PERFORMANCE CHECKLIST 14-3

MOVING THE PATIENT

		S	U	Comments
1.	Refer to medical record, care plan, or Kardex for special interventions	❑	❑	_____
2.	Assemble equipment	❑	❑	_____
3.	Wash hands	❑	❑	_____
4.	Introduce self	❑	❑	_____
5.	Identify patient	❑	❑	_____
6.	Explain procedure	❑	❑	_____
7.	Prepare patient for procedure; close doors and adjust the bed level	❑	❑	_____
8.	Arrange for assistance as necessary	❑	❑	_____
9.	Lifting and moving patient up in bed			
	a. Place patient supine with head flat	❑	❑	_____
	b. Face side of bed and provide base of support	❑	❑	_____
	c. Place one arm under axilla and opposite arm under shoulder and neck	❑	❑	_____
	d. Ask patient to flex knees and push up with feet on count of 3 while assisting	❑	❑	_____
	e. Nurses position selves on both sides of patient facing each other and support patient's back with one arm with the second arm under shoulder and neck	❑	❑	_____
	f. On count of 3, each nurse moves patient up	❑	❑	_____
	g. This may also be accomplished by using a pull sheet	❑	❑	_____
	(1) Roll patient from side to side placing a pull sheet under the patient	❑	❑	_____

		S	U	Comments
	(2) One nurse on opposite side of the patient's bed grasps pull sheet firmly with hands near patient's upper arms and hips, rolling the sheet material until hands are close to the patient	❏	❏	_____
	(3) Nurses' knees are flexed with body facing the direction of the move	❏	❏	_____
	(4) Instruct patient to rest arms on body and to lift head on the count of 3	❏	❏	_____
10.	Turning the patient			
a.	Stand with feet slightly apart and flex knees	❏	❏	_____
b.	Place one arm under patient's neck and shoulders and other arm under waist	❏	❏	_____
c.	Move patient toward nurse	❏	❏	_____
d.	Turn patient on side facing raised side rail	❏	❏	_____
e.	Flex one leg over the other, place pad or pillow between legs	❏	❏	_____
f.	Align shoulders	❏	❏	_____
g.	Support back with pillows if necessary	❏	❏	_____
h.	Assess appropriate body alignment	❏	❏	_____
11.	Dangling patient			
a.	Assess pulse and respirations	❏	❏	_____
b.	Move patient to side of bed toward nurse	❏	❏	_____
c.	Lower bed to lowest position	❏	❏	_____
d.	Raise head of bed	❏	❏	_____
e.	Support patient's shoulders and help to swing legs around and off bed	❏	❏	_____
f.	This may also be accomplished by rolling the patient onto his/her side before sitting up	❏	❏	_____

	S	**U**	**Comments**
g. Help patient don slippers; cover legs	❏	❏	_____
h. Assess patient's pulse and respirations	❏	❏	_____

12. Logrolling the patient

	S	**U**	**Comments**
a. Enlist assistance of at least one other person	❏	❏	_____
b. Lower head of bed as low as the patient can tolerate			
c. Place a pillow between the patient's legs	❏	❏	_____
d. Extend patient's arm over patient's head unless shoulder movement is restricted	❏	❏	_____
e. Both caregivers on the same side of the bed, one places one hand on the patient's shoulder and the other on the hip while the other nurse places one hand to supports the back and the other behind the knees. If a pull sheet is used, hands are placed alternately to provide even support for the length of the rolled sheet	❏	❏	_____
f. Using a count of 3, turn the patient with a continuous, smooth, coordinated effort	❏	❏	_____
g. Support the patient with pillows	❏	❏	_____

13. Transferring the patient from bed to straight chair or wheelchair

	S	**U**	**Comments**
a. Lower bed to lowest position	❏	❏	_____
b. Raise head of bed	❏	❏	_____
c. Support patient's shoulder, and help patient to sit up and to swing legs around and off of bed	❏	❏	_____
d. Assist patient to don robe and slippers	❏	❏	_____
e. Position chair beside bed with seat facing foot of bed			
(1) Lock wheels of wheelchair	❏	❏	_____

		S	U	Comments
(2)	Place straight chair against wall	❏	❏	_____
f.	Stand in front of patient, and place hands at waist level or below and allow patient to use arms and shoulders to facilitate the move	❏	❏	_____
g.	Assist patient to stand and swing around with back toward seat of chair	❏	❏	_____
h.	Help patient to sit down as nurse bends knees	❏	❏	_____
i.	Apply blanket over legs for warmth	❏	❏	_____
j.	If a transfer belt is used:			
(1)	Assist patient to a sitting position on side of bed	❏	❏	_____
(2)	Apply belt after patient is sitting	❏	❏	_____
(3)	Request patient to hold onto mattress or to place fists on the bed by the thighs	❏	❏	_____
(4)	Place patient's feet flat on the floor	❏	❏	_____
(5)	Request patient to lean forward	❏	❏	_____
(6)	Instruct patient to place his hands on nurse's shoulder	❏	❏	_____
(7)	Grasp the transfer belt on each side	❏	❏	_____
(8)	Brace your knees against the patient's knees (block patient's feet with your feet)	❏	❏	_____
(9)	Request patient to push down on the mattress and to stand on the count of 3. At the same time, lift the patient into a standing position as you straighten your knees	❏	❏	_____
(10)	Pivot the patient so he can grasp the arm rest of the chair—the back of his legs should be touching the chair	❏	❏	_____

		S	U	Comments

(11) Continue to turn the patient until he can grasp the other arm rest ❑ ❑ _____

(12) As you bend your hips and knees, gradually lower the patient into the chair ❑ ❑ _____

(13) The patient can assist by leaning forward and bending his elbows and knees. Make certain the patient's buttocks are up against the back of the chair ❑ ❑ _____

(14) Cover patient's lap and legs with a blanket ❑ ❑ _____

14. Transferring from bed to stretcher/gurney/back to bed

    a. Position bed flat and raise to the same height as gurney; lower side rails ❑ ❑ _____

    b. Cover patient with top sheet or blanket and remove linens without exposing patient ❑ ❑ _____

    c. Assess for IV line, Foley catheter, tubes, or surgical drains, and position them to avoid tension during the transfer ❑ ❑ _____

    d. Position the gurney as close to the bed as possible and lock the wheels of the bed and gurney (side rails should be lowered) ❑ ❑ _____

    e. When patient can assist, stand near side of gurney and instruct patient to move feet, then buttocks, and finally upper body to the gurney bringing cover along; be certain the patient's body is centered on the gurney ❑ ❑ _____

	S	**U**	**Comments**
f. When patient is unable to assist, place a folded sheet or bath blanket under patient so that it supports patient's head and extends to mid-thighs; roll the sheet or bath blanket close to the patient's body; assist patient to cross arms over chest; two caregivers reach over the bed to patient and two caregivers stand as close to the gurney as possible; a fifth caregiver stands at the foot to transfer the feet. Using a coordinating count of 3, all five caregivers lift the patient to the edge of the bed; with another effort, lift the patient from edge of bed to gurney (roller devices may be used)	❏	❏	_____
15. Wash hands	❏	❏	_____
16. Assess for appropriate body alignment	❏	❏	_____
17. Document procedure	❏	❏	_____

PERFORMANCE CHECKLIST 14-4

USING LIFTS FOR MOVING PATIENTS

		S	U	Comments
1.	Refer to medical record, care plan, or Kardex for special interventions	❑	❑	_____
2.	Assemble equipment	❑	❑	_____
3.	Wash hands	❑	❑	_____
4.	Introduce self	❑	❑	_____
5.	Identify patient	❑	❑	_____
6.	Explain procedure	❑	❑	_____
7.	Prepare for procedure: close doors, adjust bed level	❑	❑	_____
8.	Secure appropriate number of personnel	❑	❑	_____
9.	Place chair near bed	❑	❑	_____
10.	Appropriately place canvas seat under patient	❑	❑	_____
11.	Slide horseshoe-shaped bar under bed on one side	❑	❑	_____
12.	Lower horizontal bar appropriately	❑	❑	_____
13.	Fasten hooks on chain to openings in sling	❑	❑	_____
14.	Raise head of bed	❑	❑	_____
15.	Fold patient's arms over chest	❑	❑	_____
16.	Pump lift handle until patient is raised off bed	❑	❑	_____
17.	With steering handle, pull lift off bed and down to chair	❑	❑	_____
18.	Release valve slowly to lower patient toward chair	❑	❑	_____
19.	Close off valve and release straps	❑	❑	_____

		S	U	Comments
20.	Remove straps and hydraulic lift			
21.	Wash hands	❑	❑	_____
22.	Document procedure	❑	❑	_____
23.	Evaluate body alignment	❑	❑	_____
24.	Evaluate patient's response to movement	❑	❑	_____
25.	Do patient teaching	❑	❑	_____

PERFORMANCE CHECKLIST 17-1

BATHING THE PATIENT/ADMINISTERING A BACKRUB

		S	U	Comments
1.	Prepare for procedure	❑	❑	_____
2.	Refer to medical record, care plan, or Kardex	❑	❑	_____
3.	Introduce self	❑	❑	_____
4.	Identify patient			
5.	Explain procedure to patient	❑	❑	_____
6.	Wash hands and don clean gloves as appropriate	❑	❑	_____
7.	Prepare patient for intervention			
	a. Close door/pull curtain	❑	❑	_____
	b. Drape for procedure as appropriate	❑	❑	_____
	c. Suggest use of bedpan/urinal/bathroom	❑	❑	_____
	d. Arrange supplies	❑	❑	_____
	e. Adjust room temperature	❑	❑	_____
	f. Raise bed to comfortable working position	❑	❑	_____
8.	Bed bath			
	a. Lower side rail; position patient on side of bed closest to nurse	❑	❑	_____
	b. Loosen top linens from the foot of the bed; place bath blanket over the top linens; remove top linens appropriately	❑	❑	_____
	c. Place soiled laundry in laundry bag	❑	❑	_____
	d. Assist patient with oral hygiene	❑	❑	_____
	e. Remove patient's gown, all undergarments, and jewelry	❑	❑	_____

		S	U	Comments
f.	Raise side rail and fill water basin correctly	❏	❏	_____
g.	Remove pillow and raise head of bed	❏	❏	_____
h.	Form mitt with bath cloth; dip mitt and hand into bath water	❏	❏	_____
i.	Wash around patient's eyes; dry gently	❏	❏	_____
j.	Rinse bath cloth and finish washing face	❏	❏	_____
k.	Expose arm farthest from nurse; place towel lengthwise under patient's arm; place wash basin on towel and place patient's hands in basin of water; bathe arm; supporting arm, raise it above patient's head to bathe the axilla; rinse and dry well	❏	❏	_____
l.	Do nail care; clean under nails and file smooth; dry thoroughly	❏	❏	_____
m.	Bathe arm closest to nurse	❏	❏	_____
n.	Cover patient's chest with bath towel; fold bath blanket down to waist and wash chest with circular motion	❏	❏	_____
o.	Fold bath blanket down to pubic area, keeping chest covered with dry towel; wash abdomen, including umbilicus and skin folds; dry thoroughly	❏	❏	_____
p.	Raise side rail; empty basin appropriately	❏	❏	_____
q.	Rinse basin and wash cloth; refill basin correctly	❏	❏	_____
r.	Expose leg farthest away from nurse, keeping perineum covered; place bath towel lengthwise on bed under patient's leg; place wash basin on towel, and place patient's foot in basin	❏	❏	_____
s.	Use long, firm strokes to bathe leg; after soaking, do nail care	❏	❏	_____

		S	**U**	**Comments**

t.   Bathe other leg and foot ☐ ☐ _____

u.   Raise side rail; make sure patient is covered with bath blanket; change the water; lower side rail; if patient tolerates, position in prone or in Sims' position; place towel lengthwise on bed along back; wash and dry back from neckline down to buttocks ☐ ☐ _____

v.   Reposition patient in supine position; provide basin of water, soap, wash cloth, and towel and instruct patient to cleanse perineal area, while providing privacy ☐ ☐ _____

w.   Make certain patient is covered with blankets; raise side rail; empty basin, and wash and rinse basin; replace basin in bedside stand; place wash cloth in laundry bag for soiled linen ☐ ☐ _____

x.   Position patient in Sims' or prone position close to nurse; place towel lengthwise along patient's back; give back rub ☐ ☐ _____

y.   Assist patient into clean gown ☐ ☐ _____

z.   Place all soiled linen into laundry bag; make certain all bath equipment is clean and replaced as necessary ☐ ☐ _____

aa.   Place call light, overbed table, night stand, and telephone within easy reach ☐ ☐ _____

bb.   Position patient for comfort and provide warmth ☐ ☐ _____

cc.   Remove gloves; discard them in proper receptacle and wash hands ☐ ☐ _____

9.   Towel bath

    a.   Assemble supplies ☐ ☐ _____

    b.   Prepare patient

       (1) Remove patient's clothing and excess bedding; place patient on bath blanket, and cover patient with bath blanket ☐ ☐ _____

	S	U	Comments
(2) Cover with plastic any surgical dressing, casts, or areas that should not be wet	❑	❑	_____
(3) Fan-fold a clean bath blanket at foot of the bed	❑	❑	_____
(4) Place the patient in supine position	❑	❑	_____

c. Prepare towel

(1) Fold towel in half, top to bottom; fold in half again, side to side; then roll towel-bath towel with bath towel and wash cloth inside, beginning with folded edge	❑	❑	_____
(2) Place rolled-up towel-bath towel in plastic bag with selvage edges toward open end of bag	❑	❑	_____
(3) Draw 2000 ml of water at the correct temperature into plastic pitcher; measure 30 ml of concentrate with a pump; mix 2000 ml of water and concentrate	❑	❑	_____
(4) Pour mixture over towel in plastic bag and close bag	❑	❑	_____
(5) Knead the solution quickly into towel; position plastic bag with open end in sink and squeeze out excess water, giving added wringing twist to selvage edges of towel	❑	❑	_____

d. Bathe patient

(1) Fold bath blanket down to waist; remove warm, moist towel from plastic bag and place on patient's right or left chest with open edges up and outward	❑	❑	_____
(2) Open towel to cover entire body while removing top bath blanket; tuck towel-bath towel in and around body	❑	❑	_____
(3) Begin bathing at feet, using gentle, massaging motion correctly	❑	❑	_____

		S	**U**	**Comments**
(4)	Fold lower part of towel upward away from feet as bathing continues	❑	❑	_____
(5)	Place clean bath blanket up over patient as nurse moves upward; leave 3 inches of exposed skin between towel and bath blanket	❑	❑	_____
(6)	Wash face, neck, and ears with one of the prepared wash cloths	❑	❑	_____
(7)	Turn patient onto side	❑	❑	_____
(8)	Use prepared bath towel for back care	❑	❑	_____
(9)	Use second wash cloth for perineal care; don disposable gloves; a basin of warm water, soap, wash cloth, and towel may be necessary	❑	❑	_____
(10)	When bath is completed, remove towel and place with soiled linens in plastic laundry bag	❑	❑	_____
(11)	If top bath blanket is not soiled, fold for reuse	❑	❑	_____

10. Partial bed bath

a.	Place supplies within reach	❑	❑	_____
b.	Bathe areas patient cannot reach	❑	❑	_____
c.	Follow all steps of the bath	❑	❑	_____
d.	Change water; give care to back, skin, nails, and hair	❑	❑	_____

11. Tub bath or shower

a.	Determine whether activity is allowed	❑	❑	_____
b.	Make certain tub or shower appliance is clean; place nonskid mat on tub or shower floor and disposable mat outside of tub or shower	❑	❑	_____
c.	Assemble all items necessary for bathing	❑	❑	_____

		S	U	Comments
d.	Assist patient to tub or shower	❑	❑	_____
e.	Instruct patient on how to use call signal; place "in use" sign on tub or shower door if private bath is not being used	❑	❑	_____
f.	If tub is used, fill with warm water at correct temperature; have patient test water, then adjust temperature; instruct patient on use of faucets—which is hot and which is cold; if shower is used, turn water on and adjust temperature	❑	❑	_____
g.	Caution patient to use safety bars; discourage use of bath oil in water; check on patient q5min; do not allow to remain in tub more than 20 minutes	❑	❑	_____
h.	Return to room when patient signals and offer to wash the patient's back; knock before entering	❑	❑	_____
i.	Assist patient out of tub and with drying; observe patient for signs and symptoms of weakness; if patient complains of weakness, vertigo, or syncope, drain tub before patient gets out and place towel over patient's shoulder	❑	❑	_____
j.	Assist patient into clean gown, robe, and slippers; accompany to room, position for comfort	❑	❑	_____
k.	Return to shower or tub; clean according to agency policy; place all soiled linens in laundry bag and return all articles to patient's bedside	❑	❑	_____
l.	Wash hands	❑	❑	_____
12.	Tepid sponge bath for temperature reduction			
a.	Observe patient for elevated temperature	❑	❑	_____
b.	Explain procedure to patient	❑	❑	_____
c.	Assemble equipment	❑	❑	_____

		S	**U**	**Comments**

d.   Cover patient with bath blanket, remove gown, and close windows and doors   ❏   ❏   _____

e.   Test water temperature; place wash cloths in water, then apply wet cloths to each axilla and groin; if patient is in tub, allow to stay in water for 20–30 minutes   ❏   ❏   _____

f.   Gently sponge an extremity for about 5 minutes; if patient is in tub, gently sponge water over upper torso, chest, and back   ❏   ❏   _____

g.   Continue sponge bath to other extremities, back, and buttocks for 3–5 minutes each; determine temperature and pulse q15min   ❏   ❏   _____

h.   Change water and reapply freshly moistened wash cloths to axilla and groin as necessary   ❏   ❏   _____

i.   Continue with sponge bath until body temperature falls to slightly above normal; keep body parts that are not being sponged covered; discontinue procedure according to agency policy   ❏   ❏   _____

j.   Dry patient thoroughly and cover with light blanket or sheet; avoid rubbing the skin too vigorously; leave patient in comfortable position   ❏   ❏   _____

k.   Return equipment to storage, clean area, and change bed linens as necessary; wash hands   ❏   ❏   _____

13.   Medicated bath

a.   Prepare tub bath   ❏   ❏   _____

b.   Add agent as ordered   ❏   ❏   _____

c.   Assist patient to tub   ❏   ❏   _____

d.   Allow patient to remain in tub for required time   ❏   ❏   _____

e.   Assist patient out of tub   ❏   ❏   _____

	S	U	Comments

f. Gently pat dry; teach patient not to scratch lesions to avoid further irritation and to prevent infection ❏ ❏ _____

g. Assist patient into gown or pajamas ❏ ❏ _____

h. Assist patient to return to bed, and position for comfort ❏ ❏ _____

14. Administering the backrub

a. Lower side rail; position patient with back toward nurse and drape patient with bath blanket after top linens have been fan-folded neatly to the foot of the bed ❏ ❏ _____

b. Warm hands if necessary; warm lotion by holding some in hands; explain that lotion may feel cool ❏ ❏ _____

c. Begin massage by starting in sacral area using circular motion; stroke upwards to shoulders ❏ ❏ _____

d. Use firm, smooth strokes to massage over scapulae ❏ ❏ _____

e. Continue to upper arms with one smooth stroke and down along side of back to iliac crest ❏ ❏ _____

f. Gently but firmly knead skin by grasping area between thumb and fingers; work across each shoulder and around nape of neck; continue downward along each side to sacrum to increase circulation. Do not break contact with patient's skin ❏ ❏ _____

g. With long, smooth strokes, end massage, remove excess lubricant from patient's back with towel, and retie gown ❏ ❏ _____

h. Position for comfort; lower bed and raise side rail as needed and place call button within easy reach ❏ ❏ _____

i. Place soiled laundry in proper receptacle and wash hands ❏ ❏ _____

	S	U	Comments

15. Postprocedure

    a.   Assess patient:

        (1) Tolerance of activity   ❏   ❏ _____

        (2) Level of discomfort   ❏   ❏ _____

        (3) Cognitive ability   ❏   ❏ _____

        (4) Musculoskeletal function; extent of joint ROM   ❏   ❏ _____

        (5) Risk for skin impairment   ❏   ❏ _____

        (6) Knowledge of skin hygiene in terms of its importance   ❏   ❏ _____

        (7) Vital signs   ❏   ❏ _____

    b.   Document:

        (1) Type of bath   ❏   ❏ _____

        (2) Duration of treatment   ❏   ❏ _____

        (3) Level of assistance required   ❏   ❏ _____

        (4) Condition of skin   ❏   ❏ _____

        (5) Vital signs, if applicable   ❏   ❏ _____

        (6) Patient's response   ❏   ❏ _____

        (7) Patient teaching   ❏   ❏ _____

    c.   Report alterations in skin integrity to nurse in charge or physician   ❏   ❏ _____

PERFORMANCE CHECKLIST 17-2

ADMINISTERING ORAL HYGIENE

		S	U	Comments
1.	Prepare for procedure	❏	❏	_____
2.	Refer to medical record, care plan, or Kardex	❏	❏	_____
3.	Assemble supplies	❏	❏	_____
4.	Introduce self	❏	❏	_____
5.	Identify patient	❏	❏	_____
6.	Explain procedure to patient	❏	❏	_____
7.	Assess patient				
a.	Integrity of lips, teeth, buccal mucosa, gums, palate, and tongue	❏	❏	_____
b.	Risk of dehydration	❏	❏	_____
c.	Presence of nasogastric or oxygen (O_2) tubes	❏	❏	_____
d.	Chemotherapeutic drugs or radiation therapy to head and neck	❏	❏	_____
e.	Presence of artificial airway	❏	❏	_____
f.	Oral surgery, trauma to mouth	❏	❏	_____
g.	Aging	❏	❏	_____
h.	Diabetes mellitus	❏	❏	_____
i.	Ability to perform own oral care	❏	❏	_____
8.	Wash hands and don clean gloves	❏	❏	_____
9.	Prepare patient for intervention				
a.	Close door/pull privacy curtain	❏	❏	_____
b.	Raise bed to comfortable working position	❏	❏	_____

		S	U	Comments
c.	Arrange supplies	❏	❏	_____
d.	Position patient in semi-Fowler's	❏	❏	_____
e.	Position patient's head toward you if patient is unconscious	❏	❏	_____

10. Oral care

		S	U	Comments
a.	Place towel under patient's face and emesis basin under patient's chin	❏	❏	_____
b.	Carefully separate patient's jaws	❏	❏	_____
c.	Cleanse mouth; clean inner and outer teeth surfaces; swab roof of mouth and inside cheeks; use flashlight for better visualization of oral cavity; gently swab tongue; rinse and repeat cleansing action as necessary	❏	❏	_____
d.	Apply lubricant to lips	❏	❏	_____

11. Cleansing dentures

		S	U	Comments
a.	Fill emesis basin half full of tepid water	❏	❏	_____
b.	Ask patient to remove dentures and place in emesis basin; if patient is unable to remove own dentures, break suction that holds upper denture in place; with gauze apply gentle downward tug and carefully remove from patient's mouth; next remove lower denture	❏	❏	_____
c.	Cleanse biting surfaces; cleanse outer and inner teeth surfaces; be certain to cleanse under surface of dentures	❏	❏	_____
d.	Rinse dentures thoroughly with tepid water	❏	❏	_____
e.	Replace dentures either in patient's mouth or in container of solution placed in safe location	❏	❏	_____

		S	U	Comments

f. When reinserting the dentures, replace the upper denture first if patient has both dentures; moisten dentures for easier insertion; make certain that dentures are comfortably situated in patient's mouth before leaving the bedside ❏ ❏ _____

g. Before replacing dentures in patient's mouth or after storing dentures properly, gently brush patient's gums, tongue, and inside of cheeks and rinse thoroughly ❏ ❏ _____

12. Postprocedure

a. Dispose of gloves; clean and store supplies; wash hands ❏ ❏ _____

b. Position patient for comfort, raise side rail, and lower bed ❏ ❏ _____

c. Assess for patient comfort ❏ ❏ _____

d. Document:

(1) Procedure ❏ ❏ _____

(2) Pertinent observations ❏ ❏ _____

(3) Most facilities have flow sheets for documenting ADLs, but condition of oral cavity should be noted in nurse's notes ❏ ❏ _____

(4) Patient teaching ❏ ❏ _____

e. Report bleeding or presence of lesions to nurse in charge or physician ❏ ❏ _____

PERFORMANCE CHECKLIST 17-3

CARE OF THE HAIR, NAILS, AND FEET

	S	U	Comments
Prepare for procedure			
1. Refer to medical record, care plan, or Kardex	❏	❏	_____
2. Assemble supplies:			
a. Bed shampoo	❏	❏	_____
b. Shaving	❏	❏	_____
c. Nail and foot care	❏	❏	_____
3. Introduce self	❏	❏	_____
4. Identify patient	❏	❏	_____
5. Explain procedure	❏	❏	_____
6. Assess patient			
a. Contraindications to shampooing, shaving, or nail care	❏	❏	_____
b. Restrictions to positioning	❏	❏	_____
c. Condition of scalp, hair, nails, or feet; color and temperature of toes, feet, and fingers	❏	❏	_____
d. Ability to care for own hair, nails, and feet	❏	❏	_____
e. Knowledge of foot and nail care practices	❏	❏	_____
7. Wash hands and don clean gloves	❏	❏	_____
8. Prepare patient for intervention			
a. Close door/pull privacy curtain	❏	❏	_____
b. Raise bed to a comfortable working height	❏	❏	_____

	S	**U**	**Comments**
c. Arrange supplies at bedside or, if patient is able to perform procedure, have supplies available in the bathroom and offer assistance as needed	❏	❏	_____

9. Bed shampoo

a. Position patient close to one side of bed; place shampoo board under patient's head and wash basin at end of spout; make sure spout extends over edge of mattress	❏	❏	_____
b. Position rolled-up bath towel under patient's neck	❏	❏	_____
c. Brush and comb patient's hair; if hair is matted with blood, hydrogen peroxide is effective as a cleansing agent	❏	❏	_____
d. Obtain water in pitcher at correct temperature	❏	❏	_____
e. If patient is able, instruct patient to hold wash cloth over eyes; completely wet hair and apply small amount of shampoo	❏	❏	_____
f. Massage scalp with fingertips, not nails; shampoo hairline, back of neck, and sides of hair	❏	❏	_____
g. Rinse thoroughly and apply more shampoo, repeating steps e and f; rinse and repeat, rinsing until hair is free from shampoo	❏	❏	_____
h. Wrap dry towel around patient's head; dry patient's face, neck, and shoulders; dry hair and scalp using second towel if necessary	❏	❏	_____
i. Comb hair and/or dry with blow dryer	❏	❏	_____
j. Complete styling hair and position patient for comfort	❏	❏	_____

10. Shaving the patient

a. Assist patient to sitting position	❏	❏	_____

Student Name _____ Date _____ Instructor's Name _____

		S	**U**	**Comments**

b.   Observe face and neck ❏ ❏ _____

c.   Use shaving cream or soap ❏ ❏ _____

d.   Shave in direction hair grows; use short strokes; start with upper face and lips, and then extend to neck; if patient is able, it will help if he will hyperextend his head to help shave curved areas ❏ ❏ _____

e.   Pull skin taut with nondominant hand below the area being shaved ❏ ❏ _____

f.   Rinse razor after each stroke ❏ ❏ _____

g.   Rinse and dry face ❏ ❏ _____

h.   If patient desires, apply lotion or cologne ❏ ❏ _____

i.   Dispose of blades in sharps container ❏ ❏ _____

11. Hand and foot care

a.   Position patient in chair; place disposable mat under patient's feet ❏ ❏ _____

b.   Fill basin with water at correct temperature; place basin on disposable mat and assist patient to place feet into basin; allow to soak 10–20 minutes; rewarm water as necessary ❏ ❏ _____

c.   Place overbed table in low position in front of patient; fill emesis basin with water at 100°–110° F (43°–46° C); place basin on table and place patient's fingers in basin; allow fingernails to soak 10–20 minutes; rewarm water as necessary ❏ ❏ _____

d.   Using orangewood stick, gently clean under fingernails; with clippers, trim nails straight across and even with fingertips; with emery board, shape fingernails; push cuticles back gently with wash cloth or orangewood stick ❏ ❏ _____

e.   Don gloves and with wash cloth scrub areas of feet that are callused ❏ ❏ _____

		S	U	Comments
f.	Trim and clean toenails following step d	❑	❑	_____
g.	Apply lotion or cream to hands and feet; return patient to bed and position for comfort	❑	❑	_____
h.	On completion of procedure, observe the nails and surrounding tissue for condition of skin and any remaining rough edges	❑	❑	_____
i.	If the patient's nails are extremely hard or if the patient is unable to perform personal nail care, a podiatrist can provide nail care	❑	❑	_____

12. Postprocedure

		S	U	Comments
a.	Dispose of gloves in proper receptacle; clean and store supplies; place soiled laundry in hamper	❑	❑	_____
b.	Assess for patient's comfort, lower bed level, raise side rails, and place call button within easy reach	❑	❑	_____
c.	Document:			
(1)	Procedure	❑	❑	_____
(2)	Pertinent observations	❑	❑	_____
(3)	Most facilities have flow sheets for ADLs; shaving and nail and foot care are usually not recorded in nurse's notes; know agency policy	❑	❑	_____
(4)	Patient teaching	❑	❑	_____
d.	Report abnormal findings	❑	❑	_____

PERFORMANCE CHECKLIST 17-4

PERINEAL CARE: MALE AND FEMALE AND THE CATHETERIZED PATIENT

	S	U	Comments
Prepare for procedure			
1. Refer to medical record, care plan, or Kardex	❑	❑	_____
2. Assemble supplies:			
a. Perineal care (uncatheterized patient)	❑	❑	_____
b. Perineal care (catheterized patient)	❑	❑	_____
3. Introduce self	❑	❑	_____
4. Identify patient	❑	❑	_____
5. Explain procedure	❑	❑	_____
6. Don gloves; assess patient for:			
a. Accumulated secretions	❑	❑	_____
b. Surgical incision	❑	❑	_____
c. Lesions			
d. Ability to perform self-care	❑	❑	_____
e. Extent of care required by patient	❑	❑	_____
f. Knowledge of importance of perineal care	❑	❑	_____
7. Wash hands and don clean gloves	❑	❑	_____
8. Prepare patient for intervention			
a. Close door/pull privacy curtain	❑	❑	_____
b. Raise bed to comfortable working height and lower side rail	❑	❑	_____
c. Arrange supplies at bedside	❑	❑	_____
d. OB patients are allowed to perform this procedure by themselves while sitting on the stool by using a plastic squeeze bottle	❑	❑	_____

		S	U	Comments

e. Patients allowed tub/shower baths will do this by themselves; make certain supplies are close by

   (1) Assist patient to desired position in bed, supine for males or dorsal recumbent for females ❑ ❑ _____

   (2) Drape for procedure ❑ ❑ _____

   (3) When perineal care is given other than routinely during the bath, the nurse will need to fill the perineal bottle (peribottle) with cleansing solution and position the patient on the bedpan in bed ❑ ❑ _____

9. Female perineal care

  a. Raise side rail and fill basin two-thirds full of water at correct temperature ❑ ❑ _____

  b. Position patient in bed supine with waterproof pad/towel under buttocks; drape for privacy ❑ ❑ _____

  c. Using a disposable wash cloth wrapped around one hand, wash and dry patient's upper thighs ❑ ❑ _____

  d. Wash both labia majora and labia minora; cleanse in direction anterior to posterior; use separate corner of wash cloth for each skin fold ❑ ❑ _____

  e. Separate labia to expose the urinary meatus and vaginal orifice; wash downward toward rectum with smooth strokes; use separate corner of wash cloth for each smooth stroke ❑ ❑ _____

  f. Cleanse, rinse, and dry thoroughly (if patient is on bedpan and peribottle is used, direct flow of cleansing solution down over perineal area and dry thoroughly) ❑ ❑ _____

		S	**U**	**Comments**

g. Assist patient to side-lying position and cleanse rectal area with toilet tissue; wash area by cleansing from perineal area toward anus (several wash cloths may be needed). (Many facilitates have disposable wipes; if so, use them.) Wash, rinse, and dry thoroughly ❏ ❏ _____

10. Male perineal care

   a. Raise side rail and fill basin two-thirds full of water at the correct temperature ❏ ❏ _____

   b. Position patient supine in bed ❏ ❏ _____

   c. Gently grasp shaft of penis; retract foreskin of uncircumcised patient ❏ ❏ _____

   d. Wash tip of penis with circular motion ❏ ❏ _____

   e. Cleanse from meatus outward; two wash cloths may be necessary; wash, rinse, and dry gently ❏ ❏ _____

   f. Replace foreskin, and wash shaft of penis with a firm but gentle downward stroke ❏ ❏ _____

   g. Rinse and dry thoroughly ❏ ❏ _____

   h. Cleanse scrotum gently; cleanse carefully in underlying skin folds; rinse and dry gently ❏ ❏ _____

   i. Assist patient to a side-lying position; cleanse anal area; follow step f of female perineal care ❏ ❏ _____

11. Perineal/catheter care

   a. Raise side rail and fill basin two-thirds full of water at the correct temperature ❏ ❏ _____

   b. Position and drape the female patient in bed, supine as described in step 9 ❏ ❏ _____

   c. Cleanse around urethral meatus and adjacent catheter; cleanse entire catheter with soap and water ❏ ❏ _____

		S	U	Comments
d.	Repeat cleansing to remove all exudate from meatus and catheter	❏	❏	_____
e.	If ointment is ordered, open package of sterile cotton-tipped applicators; do not touch cotton tip; apply ointment to applicator; do not touch wrapper to cotton tip	❏	❏	_____
f.	Apply ointment to junction of catheter and urethral meatus	❏	❏	_____

12. Postprocedure

		S	U	Comments
a.	Remove gloves; clean and store equipment; dispose of contaminated supplies in proper receptacle; wash hands	❏	❏	_____
b.	Position patient for comfort	❏	❏	_____
c.	Document:			
(1)	Procedure	❏	❏	_____
(2)	Pertinent observations such as:			
	• Character and amount of discharge and odor if present	❏	❏	_____
	• Condition of genitalia	❏	❏	_____
	• Patient's ability to perform own care	❏	❏	_____
	• Patient teaching	❏	❏	_____
d.	Report abnormal findings to nurse in charge or physician	❏	❏	_____

PERFORMANCE CHECKLIST 17-5

Bedmaking

	S	U	Comments
Prepare for procedure			
1. Refer to medical record, care plan, or Kardex	❑	❑	_____
2. Assemble supplies	❑	❑	_____
3. Introduce self	❑	❑	_____
4. Identify patient	❑	❑	_____
5. Explain procedure	❑	❑	_____
6. Wash hands and don gloves	❑	❑	_____
7. Prepare patient			
a. Close door/pull privacy curtain	❑	❑	_____
b. Raise bed to appropriate height and lower side rail on the side closest to the nurse	❑	❑	_____
c. Lower head of bed if patient can tolerate it	❑	❑	_____
d. Assess patient's tolerance of procedure; be alert for signs of discomfort and fatigue	❑	❑	_____
8. Occupied bed			
a. Remove spread and blanket separately and, if soiled, place in laundry bag; if linens will be reused, fold neatly and place over back of chair	❑	❑	_____
b. Place bath blanket over patient on top of sheet	❑	❑	_____
c. Request patient to hold onto bath blanket and remove top linens	❑	❑	_____
d. Place soiled sheet in laundry bag	❑	❑	_____
e. With assistance from coworker, slide mattress to top of bed	❑	❑	_____

		S	U	Comments

f. Position patient to far side of bed with the back toward nurse; adjust pillow for comfort; be sure side rail is up ❑ ❑ _____

g. Beginning at head and moving toward foot, loosen bottom linens; fan-fold linen draw sheet, protective draw sheet, and bottom sheet, tucking edges of linens under patient ❑ ❑ _____

h. Apply clean linens to bed by first placing mattress pad (if used); fold lengthwise, making sure crease is in center of bed; likewise, unfold bottom sheet and place over mattress pad; hem of bottom sheet (if flat is used) should be placed with rough edge down and just even with bottom edge of mattress ❑ ❑ _____

i. Miter corners (if flat sheet) at head of bed; continue to tuck in sheet along side toward front, keeping linens smooth ❑ ❑ _____

j. Reach under the patient to pull out protective draw sheet (if used), and smooth out over clean bottom sheet; tuck in; unfold linen draw sheet and place center fold along middle of bed, smooth out over protective draw sheet and tuck in; tuck in folded linens in center of bed so they are under patient's buttocks and torso ❑ ❑ _____

k. Keep palms down as linens are tucked under mattress ❑ ❑ _____

l. Raise side rail and assist patient to roll slowly toward nurse over folds of linen; go to opposite side of bed and lower side rail ❑ ❑ _____

m. Loosen edges of all soiled linens; remove by folding into a bundle and place in laundry bag ❑ ❑ _____

n. Spread clean linens, including protective draw sheet, out over mattress and smooth out wrinkles; assist patient to supine position and position pillow for comfort ❑ ❑ _____

		S	U	Comments

o. Miter top corner of bottom sheet, pulling sheet taut; tuck bottom sheet under mattress all the way to foot of bed ❑ ❑ _____

p. Smooth out draw sheets; pulling sheet taut, tuck in protective draw sheet and then tuck in linen draw sheet ❑ ❑ _____

q. Place top sheet over bath blanket that is over patient; request patient to hold top sheet while nurse removes bath blanket; place blanket in laundry bag; if blanket is used, place over sheet and place spread over blanket; form cuff with top linens under patient's chin ❑ ❑ _____

r. Tuck in all linens at foot of bed, making modified miter corner; raise side rail and make opposite side of bed; make toe pleat by placing fold either lengthwise down center of bed or across foot of bed ❑ ❑ _____

s. Change pillow case; grasp closed end of pillow case, turning case inside out over hand; now grasp one end of pillow with hand in the case and smooth out wrinkles ❑ ❑ _____

9. Unoccupied bed

a. Starting at head of bed, loosen linens all the way to foot; go to opposite side of bed, loosen linens, roll all linens up in ball, and place in soiled laundry bag; wash hands after handling soiled linens ❑ ❑ _____

b. If blanket and spread are to be reused, fold neatly and place over back of chair; remove soiled pillow case ❑ ❑ _____

c. Slide mattress to head of bed ❑ ❑ _____

d. If necessary, clean mattress with cloth moistened with antiseptic solution and dry thoroughly ❑ ❑ _____

		S	U	Comments

e. Begin to make bed standing on side where lines are placed; unfold bottom sheet, placing fold lengthwise down center of bed; make certain rough edge of hem lies down away from patient's heels and even with edge of mattress; smooth out sheet over top edge of mattress and miter corners; tuck remaining sheet under mattress all the way to foot ❏ ❏ _____

f. Place draw sheet on bed so that center fold lies down middle of bed; if protective draw sheet is to be used, place it on first; smooth out over mattress and tuck in; keep palms down ❏ ❏ _____

g. Place top sheet over bed and smooth out; place blanket over top sheet; smooth out; place spread over blanket and smooth out; make cuff with top linens ❏ ❏ _____

h. Allow for toe pleat; make modified mitered corner by not tucking tip of under mattress ❏ ❏ _____

i. Move to opposite side of bed and complete making bed as described in steps 9e to 9h; pull linens tight and keep taut as linens are tucked in ❏ ❏ _____

j. Put on clean pillow case (see step 8s); position pillow at head of bed; place call light within easy reach and lower bed level ❏ ❏ _____

k. If patient is to return to bed, fan-fold top linens down to foot of bed; make sure cuff at top of linens is easily accessible to patient ❏ ❏ _____

10. Postprocedure

a. Arrange personal items on bed table or bedside stand and place within patient's easy reach ❏ ❏ _____

b. Leave area neat and clean ❏ ❏ _____

c. Place all soiled linens in proper receptacle; wash hands ❏ ❏ _____

		S	U	Comments
d.	Assist patient to bed and position for comfort	❏	❏	_____
e.	Documentation (Bedmaking does not need to be recorded. Record patient's vital signs, signs and symptoms only if there are changes.)	❏	❏	_____
f.	Report any abnormal findings to nurse in charge or physician	❏	❏	_____

PERFORMANCE CHECKLIST 17-6

POSITIONING THE BEDPAN

	S	U	Comments
Prepare for procedure			
1. Refer to medical record, care plan, or Kardex	❑	❑	_____
2. Assess patient's needs	❑	❑	_____
3. Assemble supplies	❑	❑	_____
4. Introduce self	❑	❑	_____
5. Identify patient	❑	❑	_____
6. Explain procedure	❑	❑	_____
7. Prepare patient			
a. Close door/pull privacy curtain	❑	❑	_____
b. Arrange supplies close to the bedside	❑	❑	_____
c. Place protective pad under patient's buttocks	❑	❑	_____
8. Wash hands and don clean gloves	❑	❑	_____
9. Warm metal bedpan under running warm water	❑	❑	_____
10. Position patient in supine position with knees flexed and bottom of feet flat on bed surface; as patient raises hips, support patient's lower back with arm and position bedpan under patient; when patient has finished with elimination, remove bedpan in same manner	❑	❑	_____
11. For patient unable to assist self on bedpan:			
a. Turn patient away toward opposite side rail, moving linens out of way	❑	❑	_____
b. Fit bedpan to patient's buttocks	❑	❑	_____
c. Assist patient to turn over onto bedpan while nurse secures bedpan	❑	❑	_____

		S	U	Comments
d.	Raise head of bed 30 degrees	❏	❏	_____
e.	Place toilet tissue and call light within easy reach	❏	❏	_____

12. For those patients who can be out of bed but are unable to ambulate far, there is the bedside commode

		S	U	Comments
a.	Some are equipped with wheels that allow the patient to be moved to the bathroom	❏	❏	_____
b.	When transferring a patient to the commode, assist the patient in the same manner as if assisting to a chair	❏	❏	_____

13. Postprocedure

   a. Document according to agency policy:

		S	U	Comments
(1)	Amount	❏	❏	_____
(2)	Color	❏	❏	_____
(3)	Consistency	❏	❏	_____
(4)	Abnormal findings	❏	❏	_____

	S	U	Comments
14. Report abnormal findings	❏	❏	_____

PERFORMANCE CHECKLIST 18-1

PREPARING PATIENT FOR DIAGNOSTIC EXAMINATION

		S	U	Comments
1.	Refer to medical record, care plan, or Kardex	❏	❏	_____
2.	Ensure that informed consent has been obtained when necessary	❏	❏	_____
3.	Assemble equipment and supplies	❏	❏	_____
4.	Introduce self	❏	❏	_____
5.	Identify patient	❏	❏	_____
6.	Explain procedure	❏	❏	_____
7.	Assess patient's understanding of procedure and purpose	❏	❏	_____
8.	Assess patient for allergy to the dye	❏	❏	_____
9.	Prepare patient for procedure			
	a. Transfer to examining room; maintain safety precautions	❏	❏	_____
	b. Close door and pull curtains	❏	❏	_____
	c. Raise bed or arrange examination table to convenient height	❏	❏	_____
	d. Drape for procedure	❏	❏	_____
10.	Wash hands and don clean gloves	❏	❏	_____
11.	Assist physician with procedure	❏	❏	_____

Postprocedure

		S	U	Comments
12.	Answer patient's questions	❏	❏	_____
13.	Deliver specimen to laboratory promptly, label specimen according to agency policy	❏	❏	_____
14.	Document procedure	❏	❏	_____

PERFORMANCE CHECKLIST 18-2

COLLECTING A MIDSTREAM URINE SPECIMEN

		S	U	Comments
1.	Refer to medical record, care plan, or Kardex	❏	❏	_____
2.	Assemble supplies	❏	❏	_____
3.	Introduce self	❏	❏	_____
4.	Identify patient	❏	❏	_____
5.	Explain procedure to patient; make certain patient understands how to perform procedure	❏	❏	_____
6.	Prepare patient for procedure	❏	❏	_____
7.	Close door	❏	❏	_____
8.	Offer assistance if required	❏	❏	_____
9.	Wash hands and don clean gloves	❏	❏	_____
10.	If patient is able, allow patient to cleanse perineum from anterior to posterior with antiseptic solution. Separate the labia well on a female patient. Retract foreskin of an uncircumcised male. Use each cotton ball that is saturated with antiseptic solution one time only. If patient is unable to cleanse area, the nurse will don gloves and assist with procedure	❏	❏	_____
11.	Request that patient (1) begin to void into urine receptacle about 30 ml, then place the sterile specimen container so that sides of the labia of the female do not touch; (2) without stopping flow, void a small amount into specimen cup; and (3) without stopping flow, finish voiding into toilet	❏	❏	_____
12.	Secure lid on container	❏	❏	_____
13.	Cleanse and return toilet seat collector	❏	❏	_____
14.	Remove gloves and dispose of properly	❏	❏	_____

		S	U	Comments
15.	Wash hands	❏	❏	_____
16.	Label specimen appropriately; enclose in plastic bag for transport	❏	❏	_____
17.	Ensure that specimen is taken to laboratory with requisition	❏	❏	_____
18.	Document procedure	❏	❏	_____
19.	Do patient teaching	❏	❏	_____

PERFORMANCE CHECKLIST 18-3

COLLECTING A STERILE URINE SPECIMEN VIA CATHETER PORT

		S	U	Comments
1.	Refer to medical record, care plan, or Kardex	❏	❏	_____
2.	Assemble supplies	❏	❏	_____
3.	Introduce self	❏	❏	_____
4.	Identify patient	❏	❏	_____
5.	Explain procedure to patient	❏	❏	_____
6.	Wash hands and don clean gloves	❏	❏	_____
7.	Catheter port collection:			
a.	Clamp just below catheter port for about 30 minutes	❏	❏	_____
b.	Return in 30 minutes; clean port with alcohol prep	❏	❏	_____
c.	Insert needle into port at 30-degree angle, and withdraw 5–10 ml of urine for a specimen	❏	❏	_____
d.	Place urine in sterile specimen cup	❏	❏	_____
e.	Unclamp catheter	❏	❏	_____
f.	Label specimen, enclose in plastic bag, and send to laboratory with requisition	❏	❏	_____
8.	Remove gloves and wash hands	❏	❏	_____
9.	Document procedure and observations	❏	❏	_____

Student Name _____ Date _____ Instructor's Name _____

COLLECTING A 24-HOUR URINE SPECIMEN

		S	U	Comments
1.	Refer to medical record, care plan, or Kardex	❏	❏	_____
2.	Assemble supplies and equipment	❏	❏	_____
3.	Introduce self	❏	❏	_____
4.	Identify patient	❏	❏	_____
5.	Post signs in all appropriate places	❏	❏	_____
6.	Explain procedure			
a.	Instruct patient about the importance of collecting all urine for a period of 24 hours	❏	❏	_____
b.	Instruct patient not to place toilet tissue or fecal material in urine	❏	❏	_____
7.	Wash hands	❏	❏	_____
8.	Have patient void when the 24-hour specimen collection is to begin; discard this voiding	❏	❏	_____
9.	Place labeled container on ice if required	❏	❏	_____
10.	Save all urine for the 24-hour period; place each voided specimen into the larger container with preservative	❏	❏	_____
11.	Instruct patient to void a few minutes before end of 24 hours; this urine is part of the 24-hour specimen	❏	❏	_____
12.	Send specimen to lab promptly; be certain label is complete with all pertinent information. If more than one container is necessary, make certain all are labeled and numbered	❏	❏	_____
13.	Document procedure and observations	❏	❏	_____
14.	Do patient teaching	❏	❏	_____

PERFORMANCE CHECKLIST 18-5

MEASURING BLOOD GLUCOSE LEVELS

	S	U	Comments
1. Refer to medical record, care plan, or Kardex	❏	❏	_____
2. Assemble supplies	❏	❏	_____
3. Introduce self	❏	❏	_____
4. Identify patient	❏	❏	_____
5. Explain procedure to patient	❏	❏	_____
6. Wash hands and don clean gloves	❏	❏	_____
7. Remove cap from lancet using sterile technique	❏	❏	_____
8. Place lancet into automatic lancing device according to instructions in operating manual	❏	❏	_____
9. Select site on side of any fingertip (heel used for infant)	❏	❏	_____
10. Wipe selected site with alcohol swab, and discard	❏	❏	_____
11. Ask patient to hold arm at side for 30 seconds	❏	❏	_____
12. Gently squeeze fingertip with thumb of same hand	❏	❏	_____
13. Hold lancing device	❏	❏	_____
14. Place trigger platform of lancing device on side of finger, and press	❏	❏	_____
15. Squeeze finger in downward motion (wipe off first drop of blood)	❏	❏	_____
16. While holding strip level, touch drop of blood to test pad (prevent skin from touching test pad)	❏	❏	_____
17. Begin recommended timing. After 60 seconds, blot blood off test strip, place reagent strip into appropriate site on meter, and wait for numeric readout	❏	❏	_____

	S	U	Comments
18. Remove lancet from device, and discard	❏	❏	_____
19. Remove gloves and discard; wash hands	❏	❏	_____
20. Document procedure and observations	❏	❏	_____
21. Do patient teaching	❏	❏	_____

PERFORMANCE CHECKLIST 18-6

COLLECTING A STOOL SPECIMEN

		S	U	Comments
1.	Refer to medical record, care plan, or Kardex	❏	❏	_____
2.	Assemble supplies	❏	❏	_____
3.	Introduce self	❏	❏	_____
4.	Identify patient	❏	❏	_____
5.	Explain procedure to patient; make certain patient understands what is expected	❏	❏	_____
6.	Wash hands and don gloves	❏	❏	_____
7.	Assist to bathroom when necessary	❏	❏	_____
8.	Request that patient defecate into commode, specimen device, or bedpan, and prevent urine from entering specimen	❏	❏	_____
9.	Transfer stool to specimen cup with use of a tongue blade and close lid	❏	❏	_____
10.	Remove gloves and wash hands	❏	❏	_____
11.	Attach lab slip, enclose in plastic bag, and send specimen to laboratory	❏	❏	_____
12.	Assist patient to bed	❏	❏	_____
13.	Document procedure and observations	❏	❏	_____
14.	Do patient teaching	❏	❏	_____

PERFORMANCE CHECKLIST 18-7

DETERMINING THE PRESENCE OF OCCULT BLOOD IN STOOL

		S	U	Comments
1.	Refer to medical record, care plan, or Kardex	❑	❑	_____
2.	Assemble supplies	❑	❑	_____
3.	Introduce self	❑	❑	_____
4.	Identify patient	❑	❑	_____
5.	Explain procedure to patient	❑	❑	_____
6.	Wash hands, and don gloves	❑	❑	_____
7.	Collect stool specimen appropriately	❑	❑	_____
8.	Follow steps on Hemoccult slide test			
a.	Open flap	❑	❑	_____
b.	Smear very small amount of stool with tongue blade in first box (A)	❑	❑	_____
c.	Smear very small amount of stool with tongue blade from another part of stool specimen, and transfer to box (B)	❑	❑	_____
d.	Close card, label (label before collecting specimen), and place in plastic bag	❑	❑	_____
e.	Send specimen to lab	❑	❑	_____
9.	Remove gloves and wash hands	❑	❑	_____
10.	Document procedure and observations	❑	❑	_____
11.	Do patient teaching	❑	❑	_____

PERFORMANCE CHECKLIST 18-8

COLLECTING A SPUTUM SPECIMEN

		S	U	Comments
1.	Refer to medical record, care plan, or Kardex	❏	❏	_____
2.	Assemble supplies	❏	❏	_____
3.	Introduce self	❏	❏	_____
4.	Identify patient	❏	❏	_____
5.	Explain procedure to patient	❏	❏	_____
6.	Wash hands and don gloves	❏	❏	_____
7.	Position patient in Fowler's position	❏	❏	_____
8.	Instruct patient to take three breaths, and force cough into sterile container	❏	❏	_____
9.	Label specimen container	❏	❏	_____
10.	Attach laboratory requisition, place in plastic bag, and send specimen to laboratory	❏	❏	_____
11.	Remove gloves and wash hands	❏	❏	_____
12.	Document procedure and observations	❏	❏	_____
13.	Do patient teaching	❏	❏	_____

PERFORMANCE CHECKLIST 18-9

Performing an Electrocardiogram (ECG, EKG)

		S	U	Comments
1.	Refer to medical record	❏	❏	_____
2.	Assemble supplies	❏	❏	_____
3.	Introduce self	❏	❏	_____
4.	Identify patient	❏	❏	_____
5.	Explain procedure	❏	❏	_____
6.	Assess patient for:			
	a. Chest pain	❏	❏	_____
	b. Dyspnea	❏	❏	_____
	c. Heart rate and rhythm	❏	❏	_____
	d. Blood pressure, pulse, respirations	❏	❏	_____
7.	Arrange equipment and complete necessary charges	❏	❏	_____
8.	Prepare patient for procedure:			
	a. Provide privacy	❏	❏	_____
	b. Position patient supine and provide for comfort	❏	❏	_____
	c. Drape patient	❏	❏	_____
	d. Adjust bed to proper height and lower nearest side rail	❏	❏	_____
9.	Wash hands and don clean gloves	❏	❏	_____
10.	Perform ECG:			
	a. Cleanse and wipe skin area with alcohol	❏	❏	_____
	b. Apply electrode paste and attach leads. For 12-lead ECG:			
	(1) Chest (precordial leads)			
	• V_1—Fourth intercostal space (ICS) at right sternal border	❏	❏	_____

		S	U	Comments
•	V_2—Fourth ICS at left sternal border	❑	❑	_____
•	V_3—Midway between V_2 and V_4	❑	❑	_____
•	V_4—Fifth ICS at midclavicular line	❑	❑	_____
•	V_5—Left anterior axillary line at level of V_4 horizontally	❑	❑	_____
•	V_6—Left mid-axillary line at level of V_4 horizontally	❑	❑	_____
(2)	Extremities—one at lower portion of each extremity			
•	$_aV_R$—Right wrist	❑	❑	_____
•	$_aV_L$—Left wrist	❑	❑	_____
•	$_AV_F$—Left ankle	❑	❑	_____
c.	Obtain tracing	❑	❑	_____
d.	Disconnect leads, wipe excess paste from chest	❑	❑	_____
e.	Remove gloves, dispose of appropriately and wash hands	❑	❑	_____
f.	Deliver EGG tracing promptly to laboratory or nursing unit	❑	❑	_____
11.	Assist patient to position of comfort and place needed items within easy reach	❑	❑	_____
12.	Raise side rail and lower bed to lowest position	❑	❑	_____
13.	Store supplies and equipment as is appropriate	❑	❑	_____
14.	Document procedure			
a.	Time	❑	❑	_____
b.	Test performed	❑	❑	_____
c.	Patient's response	❑	❑	_____
15.	Do patient teaching	❑	❑	_____

PERFORMANCE CHECKLIST 18-10

Performing Venipuncture

	S	U	Comments
1. Refer to medical record	❏	❏	_____
2. Assemble supplies	❏	❏	_____
3. Introduce self	❏	❏	_____
4. Identify patient	❏	❏	_____
5. Explain procedure	❏	❏	_____
6. Assess patient	❏	❏	_____
7. Arrange equipment and complete necessary charges	❏	❏	_____
8. Prepare patient for procedure			
a. Provide privacy	❏	❏	_____
b. Position supine or semi-Fowler's with arm extended to form straight line from shoulders to waist	❏	❏	_____
c. Place small pillow or towel under upper arm	❏	❏	_____
d. Adjust bed to appropriate height and lower nearest side rail	❏	❏	_____
e. Drape patient	❏	❏	_____
9. Wash hands and don clean gloves	❏	❏	_____
10. Apply tourniquet 3–4 inches above puncture site	❏	❏	_____
11. Palpate distal pulse. If pulse is not palpable, reapply tourniquet more loosely	❏	❏	_____
12. Keep tourniquet on patient no longer than 1–2 minutes. If tourniquet is left on too long, remove and assess other extremity or wait 60 seconds before reapplying	❏	❏	_____

	S	U	Comments
13. Request patient to open and close fist several times, finally leaving fist clenched	❏	❏	_____
14. Quickly assess extremity for best venipuncture site	❏	❏	_____
15. Palpate selected vein with fingers	❏	❏	_____
16. Select venipuncture site	❏	❏	_____
17. Obtain blood samples	❏	❏	_____

a.   Syringe method:

	S	U	Comments
(1) Make certain syringe with appropriate needle is securely attached	❏	❏	_____
(2) Cleanse venipuncture site with alcohol swab and allow to dry	❏	❏	_____
(3) Remove needle cover and inform patient a "stick" will be felt	❏	❏	_____
(4) Place thumb and forefinger of nondominant hand 1 inch below site and pull skin taut. Stretch skin down until vein is stabilized	❏	❏	_____
(5) Hold syringe and needle at 15- to 30-degree angle from patient's arm with bevel up	❏	❏	_____
(6) Slowly insert needle into vein	❏	❏	_____
(7) Hold syringe securely and pull back gently on plunger	❏	❏	_____
(8) Look for blood return	❏	❏	_____
(9) Obtain desired amount of blood, keeping needle stabilized	❏	❏	_____
(10) After obtaining specimen, release tourniquet	❏	❏	_____

	S	**U**	**Comments**

(11) Apply a gauze pad or alcohol swab over needle site without applying pressure, quickly but carefully withdraw needle from vein and apply pressure to puncture site ❏ ❏ _____

(12) Carefully transfer blood from syringe into vacuum tube ❏ ❏ _____

(13) Discard needle without recapping in proper receptacle ❏ ❏ _____

(14) Remove and discard gloves ❏ ❏ _____

b. Vacuum tube method:

(1) Attach double-ended needle to vacuum tube ❏ ❏ _____

(2) Have proper blood specimen tube resting inside vacuum tube without puncturing rubber stopper ❏ ❏ _____

(3) Cleanse venipuncture site properly ❏ ❏ _____

(4) Remove needle cover and inform patient "stick" will be felt ❏ ❏ _____

(5) Place thumb and forefinger of nondominant hand 1 inch below site and pull taut. Stretch skin down until vein is stabilized ❏ ❏ _____

(6) Hold vacuum tube at a 15- to 30-degree angle from arm with bevel up ❏ ❏ _____

(7) Slowly insert needle into vein ❏ ❏ _____

(8) Grasp vacuum tube securely and advance specimen tube into needle of holder ❏ ❏ _____

(9) Note flow of blood into tube ❏ ❏ _____

(10) After specimen tube is filled, grasp vacuum tube firmly and remove tube. Insert additional specimen tubes as needed ❏ ❏ _____

	S	U	Comments
(11) After last tube is filled, release tourniquet	❏	❏	_____
(12) Apply gauze pad or alcohol pad over needle site without applying pressure and quickly but carefully withdraw needle from vein, applying pressure over puncture site	❏	❏	_____
(13) Remove and discard gloves	❏	❏	_____
18. For blood obtained by syringe, transfer specimen to tubes	❏	❏	_____
19. For blood tubes containing additives, gently rotate back and forth 8–10 times	❏	❏	_____
20. Inspect puncture site for bleeding and apply adhesive tape with gauze	❏	❏	_____
21. Assess tubes for any external contamination with blood and decontaminate with alcohol, if necessary	❏	❏	_____
22. Securely attach ID label to each tube, affix proper requisition slip, and promptly transfer to lab	❏	❏	_____
23. Assist patient to position of comfort and place needed items within easy reach	❏	❏	_____
24. Raise side rail and lower bed to lowest position	❏	❏	_____
25. Store, remove, and dispose of supplies and equipment as is appropriate	❏	❏	_____
26. Document procedure	❏	❏	_____
27. Do patient teaching	❏	❏	_____

PERFORMANCE CHECKLIST 19-1

CHANGING A STERILE DRY DRESSING

	S	U	Comments
Prepare for procedure			
1. Refer to medical record, care plan, or Kardex	❑	❑	_____
2. Introduce self	❑	❑	_____
3. Identify patient			
4. Explain the procedure	❑	❑	_____
5. Assess need for and provide patient teaching	❑	❑	_____
6. Assess patient	❑	❑	_____
7. Assemble equipment and complete necessary charges	❑	❑	_____
8. Wash hands	❑	❑	_____
9. Prepare patient for intervention			
a. Close door/pull privacy curtain	❑	❑	_____
b. Raise bed to comfortable working height; lower side rail on side nearest the nurse	❑	❑	_____
c. Position and drape patient as necessary	❑	❑	_____
During the skill:			
10. Promote patient involvement as possible	❑	❑	_____
11. Assess patient's tolerance	❑	❑	_____
12. Place refuse container in convenient location away from sterile field	❑	❑	_____
13. Set up sterile field correctly	❑	❑	_____
14. Loosen tape appropriately	❑	❑	_____
15. Don clean gloves	❑	❑	_____

		S	U	Comments
16.	Remove dressing and discard correctly	❑	❑	_____
17.	Assess status of wound and wound drainage/ exudate correctly	❑	❑	_____
18.	Remove and discard soiled gloves	❑	❑	_____
19.	Wash hands and don sterile gloves	❑	❑	_____
20.	Cleanse wound and surrounding area correctly	❑	❑	_____
21.	Use sterile 4 × 4" dressing to dry in same manner or allow antiseptic to air dry	❑	❑	_____
22.	Cleanse drain site appropriately if applicable	❑	❑	_____
23.	Apply antibiotic ointment, if ordered, using same techniques as for cleansing	❑	❑	_____
24.	Cover wound with appropriately sized dry sterile dressing and use drain dressing, if applicable	❑	❑	_____
25.	Secure dressing with appropriate tape, Montgomery straps, or binder	❑	❑	_____

Postprocedure

		S	U	Comments
26.	Assist patient to a position of comfort and place needed items within easy reach; be certain patient has a means to call for assistance and knows how to use it	❑	❑	_____
27.	Raise the side rails and lower the bed to the lowest position	❑	❑	_____
28.	Remove gloves and all protective barriers; remove and dispose of soiled supplies and equipment appropriately	❑	❑	_____
29.	Wash hands after patient contact and after removing gloves	❑	❑	_____
30.	Document and do patient teaching	❑	❑	_____
31.	Report any unexpected appearance of wound or drainage or accidental removal of drain within an hour to physician	❑	❑	_____

PERFORMANCE CHECKLIST 19-2

APPLYING A WET-TO-DRY DRESSING

	S	U	Comments
Prepare for procedure			
1. Refer to medical record, care plan, or Kardex	❏	❏	_____
2. Introduce self	❏	❏	_____
3. Identify patient	❏	❏	_____
4. Explain the procedure	❏	❏	_____
5. Assess need for and provide patient teaching during procedure	❏	❏	_____
6. Assess patient	❏	❏	_____
7. Wash hands	❏	❏	_____
8. Assemble equipment and complete necessary charges	❏	❏	_____
9. Prepare patient for intervention			
a. Close door/pull privacy curtain	❏	❏	_____
b. Raise bed to comfortable working height; lower side rail on side nearest the nurse	❏	❏	_____
c. Position and drape patient as necessary	❏	❏	_____
During the skill:			
10. Promote patient involvement as possible	❏	❏	_____
11. Assess patient's tolerance	❏	❏	_____
12. Place waterproof pad appropriately	❏	❏	_____
13. Place refuse container appropriately	❏	❏	_____
14. Set up sterile field	❏	❏	_____
15. Loosen tape correctly	❏	❏	_____

	S	U	Comments
16. Don clean gloves; remove dressing appropriately and discard	❏	❏	_____
17. Assess status of wound and wound exudate/drainage	❏	❏	_____
18. Remove gloves and discard; wash hands and don sterile gloves	❏	❏	_____
19. Cleanse wound correctly	❏	❏	_____
20. Place 4 × 4" dressing into basin	❏	❏	_____
21. Wring excess solution from dressing, leaving it slightly moist	❏	❏	_____
22. Place dressing over open wound surfaces and press into depressed areas	❏	❏	_____
23. Apply dry dressing over wet dressing	❏	❏	_____
24. Cover with additional dressing as needed	❏	❏	_____
25. Secure with tape or Montgomery straps	❏	❏	_____

Postprocedure

	S	U	Comments
26. Assist patient to a position of comfort and place needed items within easy reach; be certain patient has a means to call for assistance and knows how to use it	❏	❏	_____
27. Raise the side rails and lower the bed to the lowest position	❏	❏	_____
28. Remove gloves and all protective barriers and dispose of soiled supplies and equipment appropriately	❏	❏	_____
29. Wash hands after patient contact and after removing gloves	❏	❏	_____
30. Document and do patient teaching	❏	❏	_____
31. Discuss change in dressing procedure with physician as wound surface becomes clean and granulation tissue is evident	❏	❏	_____

PERFORMANCE CHECKLIST 19-3

APPLYING A TRANSPARENT DRESSING

	S	U	Comments
Prepare for procedure			
1. Refer to medical record, care plan, or Kardex	❏	❏	_____
2. Introduce self	❏	❏	_____
3. Identify patient	❏	❏	_____
4. Explain procedure	❏	❏	_____
5. Assess need for and provide patient teaching during procedure	❏	❏	_____
6. Assess patient	❏	❏	_____
7. Assemble equipment and complete necessary charges	❏	❏	_____
8. Wash hands	❏	❏	_____
9. Prepare patient for intervention:			
a. Provide privacy	❏	❏	_____
b. Raise bed to working height and lower nearest side rail	❏	❏	_____
c. Position and drape patient as necessary	❏	❏	_____
During skill:			
10. Promote patient involvement as possible	❏	❏	_____
11. Assess patient's tolerance	❏	❏	_____
12. Place refuse container in convenient location away from contamination	❏	❏	_____
13. Set up sterile field	❏	❏	_____
14. Don clean gloves	❏	❏	_____
15. Loosen tape and remove old dressings	❏	❏	_____

		S	U	Comments
16.	Remove soiled gloves and with soiled dressings dispose of in refuse container	❑	❑	_____
17.	Assess status of wound	❑	❑	_____
18.	Don sterile gloves	❑	❑	_____
19.	Cleanse area gently	❑	❑	_____
20.	Allow skin surface to dry	❑	❑	_____
21.	Apply transparent dressings according to manufacturer's direction	❑	❑	_____
22.	Remove soiled gloves and discard; wash hands	❑	❑	_____

Postprocedure

		S	U	Comments
23.	Assist patient to a position of comfort and place needed items within easy reach	❑	❑	_____
24.	Raise side rail and lower bed to lowest level	❑	❑	_____
25.	Store, remove, and dispose of soiled supplies and equipment appropriately	❑	❑	_____
26.	Wash hands after patient contact	❑	❑	_____
27.	Document	❑	❑	_____
28.	Report any unexpected appearance of the wound or exudate	❑	❑	_____
29.	Do patient teaching	❑	❑	_____

PERFORMANCE CHECKLIST 19-4

PERFORMING STERILE IRRIGATION

	S	U	Comments
Prepare for procedure			
1. Refer to medical record, care plan, or Kardex for special interventions	❑	❑	_____
2. Introduce self	❑	❑	_____
3. Identify patient	❑	❑	_____
4. Explain the procedure	❑	❑	_____
5. Assess need for and provide patient teaching during procedure	❑	❑	_____
6. Assess patient	❑	❑	_____
7. Wash hands	❑	❑	_____
8. Assemble equipment and complete necessary charges	❑	❑	_____
9. Prepare patient for intervention			
a. Close door/pull privacy curtain	❑	❑	_____
b. Raise bed to comfortable working height; lower side rail on side nearest the nurse	❑	❑	_____
c. Position and drape patient as necessary	❑	❑	_____
During the skill:			
10. Promote patient involvement as possible	❑	❑	_____
11. Assess patient's tolerance	❑	❑	_____
12. Position waterproof pad appropriately	❑	❑	_____
13. Place refuse container in convenient location away from contamination	❑	❑	_____
14. Set up sterile field	❑	❑	_____

		S	U	Comments
15.	Don gown and goggles as appropriate	❏	❏	_____
16.	Don clean gloves, remove dressing, and discard appropriately	❏	❏	_____
17.	Remove gloves, dispose of in proper receptacle, and wash hands	❏	❏	_____
18.	Assess status of wound and exudate/drainage	❏	❏	_____
19.	Place collection basin appropriately	❏	❏	_____
20.	Wash hands and don sterile gloves	❏	❏	_____
21.	Cleanse area around wound correctly	❏	❏	_____
22.	Fill irrigating syringe with solution; attach soft catheter if irrigating a deep wound with small opening	❏	❏	_____
23.	Instill solution gently into wound, holding syringe approximately 1 inch above wound; if using catheter, gently insert into wound opening until slight resistance is met, pull back, and gently instill solution	❏	❏	_____
24.	Allow solution to flow from clean area of wound to dirty area	❏	❏	_____
25.	Pinch off catheter during withdrawal from wound	❏	❏	_____
26.	Refill syringe and continue irrigation until solution returns clear	❏	❏	_____
27.	Blot wound edges with sterile dressing	❏	❏	_____
28.	Redress wound, if applicable	❏	❏	_____
29.	Remove and dispose of gloves	❏	❏	_____
30.	Wash hands	❏	❏	_____

Postprocedure

| 31. | Assist patient to a position of comfort and place needed items within easy reach; be certain patient has a means to call for assistance and knows how to use it | ❏ | ❏ | _____ |

	S	U	Comments
32. Raise the side rails and lower the bed to the lowest position	❏	❏	_____
33. Store or remove and dispose of soiled supplies and equipment appropriately	❏	❏	_____
34. Wash hands after patient contact	❏	❏	_____
35. Document and do patient teaching	❏	❏	_____
36. Report immediately any evidence of fresh bleeding, sharp increase in pain, retention of irrigant, or signs of shock to attending physician	❏	❏	_____

PERFORMANCE CHECKLIST 19-5

REMOVING STAPLES OR SUTURES

	S	U	Comments
Prepare for procedure			
1. Refer to medical record, care plan, or Kardex	❏	❏	_____
2. Introduce self	❏	❏	_____
3. Identify patient	❏	❏	_____
4. Explain the procedure	❏	❏	_____
5. Assess need for and provide patient teaching during procedure	❏	❏	_____
6. Assess patient	❏	❏	_____
7. Wash hands	❏	❏	_____
8. Assemble equipment and complete necessary charges	❏	❏	_____
9. Prepare patient for intervention			
a. Close door/pull privacy curtain	❏	❏	_____
b. Raise bed to comfortable working height; lower side rail on side nearest the nurse	❏	❏	_____
c. Position and drape patient as necessary	❏	❏	_____
During the skill:			
10. Promote patient involvement as possible	❏	❏	_____
11. Assess patient's tolerance, being alert for signs and symptoms of discomfort and fatigue	❏	❏	_____
12. Place refuse container in convenient location away from sterile field	❏	❏	_____
13. Set up sterile field	❏	❏	_____
14. Don clean gloves	❏	❏	_____

	S	U	Comments
15. Remove dressing and soiled gloves; discard appropriately	❏	❏	_____
16. Assess status of wound and drainage on dressing correctly	❏	❏	_____
17. Wash hands and don sterile gloves	❏	❏	_____
18. Cleanse area correctly	❏	❏	_____

Staple removal

19. Place staple remover under both sides of staple; squeeze handles together and gently remove staples from skin	❏	❏	_____
20. Release handles and discard staple in refuse container	❏	❏	_____
21. Repeat steps 18 and 19 until all staples have been removed	❏	❏	_____
22. Count number of staples removed	❏	❏	_____
23. Notify physician immediately if inadequate wound healing is noted; discontinue removal of all staples	❏	❏	_____

Applying Steri-strips

24. It is common to see wounds closed with Steri-strips; these interventions should be followed when applying Steri-strips:

a. Gently cleanse suture line	❏	❏	_____
b. Carefully inspect the incision	❏	❏	_____
c. When skin is dry, apply Steri-strips	❏	❏	_____
d. Instruct patient to take showers rather than soak in bathtub according to physician's preference	❏	❏	_____
e. Many physicians request upon removal of sutures that only 1–3 sutures be removed at a time; Steri-strips are then applied, repeating this action until all sutures are removed and Steri-strips applied	❏	❏	_____

		S	U	Comments
25.	Assess healing status of wound	❏	❏	_____
26.	Cleanse area with antiseptic swabs	❏	❏	_____

Removal of intermittent sutures

		S	U	Comments
27.	Grasp and elevate knotted end of suture with hemostat or forceps	❏	❏	_____
28.	Snip suture at skin level on opposite side, proximal to knot	❏	❏	_____
29.	Gently remove entire suture with forceps and discard on sterile gauze	❏	❏	_____
30.	Repeat steps 26 to 28 until all sutures have been removed	❏	❏	_____

Removal of continuous sutures including blanket stitch sutures

		S	U	Comments
31.	Cut first suture close to skin on side away from knot	❏	❏	_____
32.	Remove gently from knotted side with forceps and discard on sterile gauze	❏	❏	_____
33.	Snip second suture on same side	❏	❏	_____
34.	Repeat steps 30 to 32 until all sutures have been removed	❏	❏	_____
35.	Apply sterile dressing or leave open to air as ordered	❏	❏	_____
36.	Remove gloves and wash hands	❏	❏	_____

Postprocedure

		S	U	Comments
37.	Assist patient to a position of comfort and place needed items within easy reach; be certain patient has a means to call for assistance and knows how to use it	❏	❏	_____
38.	Raise the side rails and lower the bed to the lowest position	❏	❏	_____
39.	Store or remove and dispose of soiled supplies and equipment appropriately	❏	❏	_____

		S	U	Comments
40.	Wash hands after patient contact	❏	❏	_____
41.	Document and do patient teaching	❏	❏	_____
42.	Report any abnormalities	❏	❏	_____

PERFORMANCE CHECKLIST 19-6

MAINTAINING HEMOVAC/DAVOL SUCTION AND T-TUBE DRAINAGE

		S	U	Comments
Prepare for procedure				
1.	Refer to medical record, care plan, or Kardex	❑	❑	_____
2.	Introduce self	❑	❑	_____
3.	Identify patient	❑	❑	_____
4.	Explain the procedure	❑	❑	_____
5.	Assess need for and provide patient teaching	❑	❑	_____
6.	Assess patient	❑	❑	_____
7.	Wash hands	❑	❑	_____
8.	Assemble equipment and complete necessary charges	❑	❑	_____
Prepare patient for intervention				
9.	Close door/pull privacy curtain	❑	❑	_____
10.	Raise bed to comfortable working height; lower side rail on side nearest the nurse	❑	❑	_____
11.	Position and drape patient as necessary	❑	❑	_____
During the skill:				
12.	Promote patient involvement as possible	❑	❑	_____
13.	Assess patient's tolerance	❑	❑	_____
14.	Examine drainage system	❑	❑	_____
15.	Don goggles as appropriate	❑	❑	_____
16.	Don clean gloves	❑	❑	_____
17.	Remove Hemovac/Davol plug labeled "pouring spout;" empty drainage into measuring device, handling device correctly	❑	❑	_____

	S	U	Comments
18. Hold pump of Hemovac tightly compressed and reinsert plug; when caring for a Davol, repump to reestablish suction	❏	❏	_____
19. T-tube maintenance			
a. Remove plug, holding drainage spout over calibrated container	❏	❏	_____
b. Empty drainage into measuring container and replace plug, maintaining sterility	❏	❏	_____
c. Always keep drainage bag below the level of the common bile duct to prevent contamination from backflow; may be fastened to patient's gown. Be very careful to prevent tension on and displacement of T-tube	❏	❏	_____
20. Observe the drainage	❏	❏	_____
21. Measure and record amount of drainage; rinse measuring container	❏	❏	_____
22. Position drainage system on bed and secure system	❏	❏	_____
23. Dispose of drainage and rinse measuring container	❏	❏	_____

Postprocedure

	S	U	Comments
24. Remove gloves and all protective barriers and dispose of all waste appropriately	❏	❏	_____
25. Wash hands after patient contact	❏	❏	_____
26. Assist patient to a position of comfort and place needed items within easy reach; be certain patient has a means to call for assistance and knows how to use it	❏	❏	_____
27. Raise the side rails and lower the bed to the lowest position	❏	❏	_____
28. If specimen is ordered, label and send to laboratory	❏	❏	_____
29. Wash hands after patient contact	❏	❏	_____

	S	**U**	**Comments**
30. Observe Davol/Hemovac/T-tube every 2–4 hours; measure drainage	❏	❏	_____
31. Document and do patient teaching	❏	❏	_____
32. Report any abnormal characteristics of drainage. Normal amounts of bile drainage vary from 250–500 ml for 24 hours; normal characteristics are thick consistency with greenish-brown color, slightly blood-tinged in the first 24 hours (excessive bile leakage from wound can indicate an occluded system; notify physician)	❏	❏	_____

PERFORMANCE CHECKLIST 19-7

APPLYING A BANDAGE

	S	U	Comments

Prepare for procedure

1. Refer to medical record, care plan, or Kardex ❏ ❏ _____

2. Introduce self ❏ ❏ _____

3. Identify patient ❏ ❏ _____

4. Explain the procedure ❏ ❏ _____

5. Assess need for and provide patient teaching during procedure ❏ ❏ _____

6. Assess patient ❏ ❏ _____

7. Wash hands ❏ ❏ _____

8. Assemble equipment and complete necessary charges ❏ ❏ _____

9. Prepare patient for intervention

    a. Close door/pull privacy curtain ❏ ❏ _____

    b. Raise bed to comfortable working height; lower side rail on side nearest the nurse ❏ ❏ _____

    c. Position and drape patient as necessary ❏ ❏ _____

During the skill:

10. Promote patient involvement as possible ❏ ❏ _____

11. Assess patient's tolerance ❏ ❏ _____

12. Ensure that skin and/or dressing is clean and dry ❏ ❏ _____

13. Separate any adjacent skin surfaces ❏ ❏ _____

14. Don gloves as necessary ❏ ❏ _____

15. Align part to be bandaged appropriately ❏ ❏ _____

		S	U	Comments
16.	Apply bandage from distal to proximal part	❑	❑	_____
17.	Apply bandage correctly			
	a. Circular bandage	❑	❑	_____
	b. Spiral bandage	❑	❑	_____
	c. Spiral-reverse bandage	❑	❑	_____
	d. Recurrent (stump) bandage	❑	❑	_____
	e. Figure-eight bandage	❑	❑	_____
18.	Secure first bandage before applying additional rolls	❑	❑	_____
19.	Apply additional rolls without leaving any uncovered areas	❑	❑	_____
20.	Assess tension of bandage and circulation of extremity	❑	❑	_____

Postprocedure

		S	U	Comments
21.	Assist patient to a position of comfort and place needed items within easy reach; be certain patient has a means to call for assistance and knows how to use it	❑	❑	_____
22.	Raise the side rails and lower the bed to the lowest position	❑	❑	_____
23.	Remove gloves if worn and all protective barriers; store or remove and dispose of soiled supplies and equipment appropriately	❑	❑	_____
24.	Wash hands after patient contact and after removing gloves	❑	❑	_____
25.	Document and do patient teaching	❑	❑	_____
26.	Report any unexpected outcomes	❑	❑	_____

PERFORMANCE CHECKLIST 19-8

APPLYING A BINDER, ARM SLING, AND T-BINDER

		S	U	Comments
Prepare for procedure				
1.	Refer to medical record, care plan, or Kardex	❏	❏	_____
2.	Introduce self	❏	❏	_____
3.	Identify patient	❏	❏	_____
4.	Explain the procedure	❏	❏	_____
5.	Assess need for and provide patient teaching during procedure	❏	❏	_____
6.	Assess patient	❏	❏	_____
7.	Wash hands	❏	❏	_____
8.	Assemble equipment and complete necessary charges	❏	❏	_____
9.	Prepare patient for intervention			
a.	Close door/pull privacy curtain	❏	❏	_____
b.	Raise bed to comfortable working height; lower side rail on side nearest the nurse	❏	❏	_____
c.	Position and drape patient as necessary	❏	❏	_____
During the skill:				
10.	Promote patient involvement as possible	❏	❏	_____
11.	Assess patient's tolerance	❏	❏	_____
12.	Don gloves as necessary	❏	❏	_____
13.	Change dressing if appropriate; cleanse skin if needed	❏	❏	_____
14.	Separate skin surfaces or pad bony prominences	❏	❏	_____
15.	**Apply binder**	❏	❏	_____

		S	U	Comments

a. Triangular binder (sling)

(1) Have patient flex arm at approximately 80-degree angle, depending on purpose of binder ❏ ❏ _____

(2) Place end of triangular binder over shoulder of the uninjured side ❏ ❏ _____

(3) Grasp other end of binder and bring it up and over injured arm to shoulder of injured arm ❏ ❏ _____

(4) Use square knot to tie two ends together at lateral area of neck on uninjured side ❏ ❏ _____

(5) Support wrist well with binder; do not allow it to extend over end of binder ❏ ❏ _____

(6) Fold third triangle end neatly around elbow and secure with safety pins ❏ ❏ _____

b. T-binder

(1) Using appropriate binder, place the waistband smoothly under patient's waist; tail(s) should be under patient ❏ ❏ _____

(2) Secure two ends of waistband together with safety pin ❏ ❏ _____

(3) Single tail—bring the tail up between legs to secure dressing in place; two tails—bring tails up one on each side of penis or large dressing ❏ ❏ _____

(4) Bring tails under and over waistband; secure with safety pins ❏ ❏ _____

c. Elastic abdominal binder

(1) Center binder smoothly under appropriate part of patient ❏ ❏ _____

(2) Bring ends around patient and overlap away from incision ❏ ❏ _____

PERFORMANCE CHECKLIST 19-8

APPLYING A BINDER, ARM SLING, AND T-BINDER

		S	U	Comments
Prepare for procedure				
1.	Refer to medical record, care plan, or Kardex	❏	❏	_____
2.	Introduce self	❏	❏	_____
3.	Identify patient	❏	❏	_____
4.	Explain the procedure	❏	❏	_____
5.	Assess need for and provide patient teaching during procedure	❏	❏	_____
6.	Assess patient	❏	❏	_____
7.	Wash hands	❏	❏	_____
8.	Assemble equipment and complete necessary charges	❏	❏	_____
9.	Prepare patient for intervention			
	a. Close door/pull privacy curtain	❏	❏	_____
	b. Raise bed to comfortable working height; lower side rail on side nearest the nurse	❏	❏	_____
	c. Position and drape patient as necessary	❏	❏	_____
During the skill:				
10.	Promote patient involvement as possible	❏	❏	_____
11.	Assess patient's tolerance	❏	❏	_____
12.	Don gloves as necessary	❏	❏	_____
13.	Change dressing if appropriate; cleanse skin if needed	❏	❏	_____
14.	Separate skin surfaces or pad bony prominences	❏	❏	_____
15.	**Apply binder**	❏	❏	_____

	S	U	Comments

a. Triangular binder (sling)

(1) Have patient flex arm at approximately 80-degree angle, depending on purpose of binder ❑ ❑ _____

(2) Place end of triangular binder over shoulder of the uninjured side ❑ ❑ _____

(3) Grasp other end of binder and bring it up and over injured arm to shoulder of injured arm ❑ ❑ _____

(4) Use square knot to tie two ends together at lateral area of neck on uninjured side ❑ ❑ _____

(5) Support wrist well with binder; do not allow it to extend over end of binder ❑ ❑ _____

(6) Fold third triangle end neatly around elbow and secure with safety pins ❑ ❑ _____

b. T-binder

(1) Using appropriate binder, place the waistband smoothly under patient's waist; tail(s) should be under patient ❑ ❑ _____

(2) Secure two ends of waistband together with safety pin ❑ ❑ _____

(3) Single tail—bring the tail up between legs to secure dressing in place; two tails—bring tails up one on each side of penis or large dressing ❑ ❑ _____

(4) Bring tails under and over waistband; secure with safety pins ❑ ❑ _____

c. Elastic abdominal binder

(1) Center binder smoothly under appropriate part of patient ❑ ❑ _____

(2) Bring ends around patient and overlap away from incision ❑ ❑ _____

	S	U	Comments
(3) Secure binder with Velcro or safety pins placed horizontally on abdomen	❏	❏	_____
d. For postsurgical application of scultetus abdominal binder, proceed upward from the bottom	❏	❏	_____
16. Note comfort level of patient and smooth binder to prevent wrinkles	❏	❏	_____

Postprocedure

	S	U	Comments
17. Assist patient to a position of comfort and place needed items within easy reach; be certain patient has a means to call for assistance and knows how to use it	❏	❏	_____
18. Raise the side rails and lower the bed to the lowest position	❏	❏	_____
19. Remove gloves if worn and all protective barriers; store or remove and dispose of soiled supplies and equipment appropriately	❏	❏	_____
20. Wash hands after patient contact and after removing gloves	❏	❏	_____
21. Document and do patient teaching	❏	❏	_____
22. Report any unexpected outcomes	❏	❏	_____

PERFORMANCE CHECKLIST 19-9

EYE IRRIGATION

		S	U	Comments
Prepare for procedure				
1.	Refer to medical record, care plan, or Kardex	❑	❑	_____
2.	Introduce self	❑	❑	_____
3.	Identify patient	❑	❑	_____
4.	Explain the procedure	❑	❑	_____
5.	Assess need for and provide patient teaching during procedure	❑	❑	_____
6.	Assess patient	❑	❑	_____
7.	Wash hands	❑	❑	_____
8.	Assemble equipment and complete necessary charges	❑	❑	_____
9.	Prepare patient for intervention			
	a. Close door/pull privacy curtain	❑	❑	_____
	b. Raise bed to comfortable working height; lower side rail on side nearest the nurse	❑	❑	_____
	c. Position and drape patient as necessary	❑	❑	_____
During the skill:				
10.	Promote patient involvement as possible	❑	❑	_____
11.	Assess patient's tolerance	❑	❑	_____
12.	Assess condition of both eyes	❑	❑	_____
13.	Place patient lying toward side to be irrigated	❑	❑	_____
14.	Place towel under patient's head	❑	❑	_____
15.	Use a sterile plastic squeeze bottle unless very large amounts of solutions are needed (sometimes a medicine dropper is sufficient)	❑	❑	_____

	S	U	Comments
16. Don gloves	❑	❑	_____
17. Place an emesis basin at side of face	❑	❑	_____
18. Using the thumb and index finger of the nondominant hand, separate the patient's eyelids	❑	❑	_____
19. Gently direct the irrigating solution along the conjunctiva from the inner to the outer canthus	❑	❑	_____
20. Avoid directing a forceful stream onto the eyeball	❑	❑	_____
21. Avoid touching any parts of the eye with irrigation equipment	❑	❑	_____
22. A piece of gauze may be wrapped around the gloved index finger to raise upper lid	❑	❑	_____
23. Gently dry the eyelids	❑	❑	_____
24. Remove gloves and wash hands	❑	❑	_____

Postprocedure

	S	U	Comments
25. Assist patient to a position of comfort and place needed items within easy reach; be certain patient has a means to call for assistance and knows how to use it	❑	❑	_____
26. Raise the side rails and lower the bed to the lowest position	❑	❑	_____
27. Store or remove and dispose of soiled supplies and equipment appropriately	❑	❑	_____
28. Wash hands after patient contact	❑	❑	_____
29. Document and do patient teaching	❑	❑	_____
30. Report any unexpected outcomes	❑	❑	_____

PERFORMANCE CHECKLIST 19-10

APPLICATION OF WARM, MOIST EYE COMPRESSES

		S	U	Comments
Prepare for procedure				
1.	Refer to medical record, care plan, or Kardex	❏	❏	_____
2.	Introduce self	❏	❏	_____
3.	Identify patient	❏	❏	_____
4.	Explain the procedure	❏	❏	_____
5.	Assess need for and provide patient teaching during procedure	❏	❏	_____
6.	Assess patient	❏	❏	_____
7.	Wash hands	❏	❏	_____
8.	Assemble equipment and complete necessary charges	❏	❏	_____
9.	Prepare patient for intervention			
a.	Close door/pull privacy curtain	❏	❏	_____
b.	Raise bed to comfortable working height; lower side rail on side nearest the nurse	❏	❏	_____
c.	Position and drape patient as necessary	❏	❏	_____
During the skill:				
10.	Promote patient involvement as possible	❏	❏	_____
11.	Assess patient's tolerance	❏	❏	_____
12.	Don clean gloves	❏	❏	_____
13.	Assess condition of both eyes	❏	❏	_____
14.	Assist patient to a comfortable position; when applying warm compresses, have the patient sit if possible; support the head with a pillow and turn the head slightly to the unaffected side	❏	❏	_____

		S	U	Comments
15.	Place the towel/waterproof pad under the patient's head	❏	❏	_____
16.	Use sterile technique when infection or ulceration is present; clean technique may be used for allergic reactions	❏	❏	_____
17.	Change gloves, dispose of in proper receptacle, and wash hands before treating each eye	❏	❏	_____
18.	Temperature of compresses should not exceed 120° F (49° C); to heat solution, place the uncapped bottle of solution in a basin of hot water; pour the warmed solution into a sterile bowl, filling it halfway; place sterile gauze pads in the bowl	❏	❏	_____
19.	Take two 4 × 4 gauze pads from the basin; squeeze out excess moisture	❏	❏	_____
20.	Instruct the patient to close his or her eyes; gently apply the pads—one on top of the other—to the affected eye	❏	❏	_____
21.	Do not exert pressure on eyelids	❏	❏	_____
22.	Change compress every few minutes, as necessary, for the prescribed length of time	❏	❏	_____
23.	If sterility is not necessary, moist heat may be applied by means of a clean wash cloth	❏	❏	_____
24.	After removing each compress, assess the periorbital skin for signs that the compress solution is too hot	❏	❏	_____
25.	Cleanse patient's eye and dry with the remaining gauze pads	❏	❏	_____
26.	If ordered, apply ophthalmic ointment or eye patch	❏	❏	_____

Postprocedure

27.	Assist patient to a position of comfort and place needed items within easy reach; be certain patient has a means to call for assistance and knows how to use it	❏	❏	_____

	S	**U**	**Comments**
28. Raise the side rails and lower the bed to the lowest position	❏	❏	_____
29. Remove gloves and all protective barriers; store or remove and dispose of soiled supplies and equipment appropriately	❏	❏	_____
30. Wash hands after patient contact and after removing gloves	❏	❏	_____
31. Document and do patient teaching	❏	❏	_____
32. Report any unexpected outcomes	❏	❏	_____

PERFORMANCE CHECKLIST 19-11

EAR IRRIGATIONS

		S	U	Comments
Prepare for procedure				
1.	Refer to medical record, care plan, or Kardex	❏	❏	_____
2.	Introduce self	❏	❏	_____
3.	Identify patient	❏	❏	_____
4.	Explain the procedure	❏	❏	_____
5.	Assess need for and provide patient teaching during procedure	❏	❏	_____
6.	Assess patient	❏	❏	_____
7.	Wash hands	❏	❏	_____
8.	Assemble equipment and complete necessary charges	❏	❏	_____
9.	Prepare patient for intervention			
	a. Close door/pull privacy curtain	❏	❏	_____
	b. Raise bed to comfortable working height; lower side rail on side nearest the nurse	❏	❏	_____
	c. Position and drape patient as necessary	❏	❏	_____
During the skill:				
10.	Promote patient involvement as possible	❏	❏	_____
11.	Assess patient's tolerance	❏	❏	_____
12.	Advise patient of sensations that might be experienced: vertigo, fullness, and warmth	❏	❏	_____
13.	Don gloves as necessary	❏	❏	_____
14.	Assess condition of external ear structures and canal for erythema, edema, and exudate	❏	❏	_____

	S	U	Comments
15. Assist patient to either a side-lying or sitting position with head tilted toward affected ear and position emesis basin under ear	❏	❏	_____
16. Place towel under patient's shoulder just under ear and emesis basin	❏	❏	_____
17. Inspect auditory canal for any accumulation of cerumen or debris; remove with cotton visually and with otoscope applicator and solution	❏	❏	_____
18. Assess irrigation solution for proper temperature; test temperature of solution by sprinkling a few drops of solution on inner wrist; fill bulb syringe with appropriate volume	❏	❏	_____
19. Straighten auditory canal for introduction of solution correctly according to age	❏	❏	_____
20. With tip of syringe just above canal, irrigate gently by creating steady flow of solution against roof of canal; do not occlude canal with tip of syringe	❏	❏	_____
21. Continue irrigation until all debris has been removed or all solution has been used; reassess auditory canal with otoscope	❏	❏	_____
22. Assess patient for vertigo or nausea; onset of symptoms may require temporary cessation of procedure	❏	❏	_____
23. Dry off auricle and apply cotton ball loosely to auditory meatus	❏	❏	_____
24. Position patient on side of affected ear for 10 minutes	❏	❏	_____
25. Return to patient to assess character and amount of drainage and determine patient's level of comfort	❏	❏	_____

Postprocedure

26. Assist patient to a position of comfort and place needed items within easy reach; be certain patient has a means to call for assistance and knows how to use it	❏	❏	_____

		S	U	Comments
27.	Raise the side rails and lower the bed to the lowest position	❏	❏	_____
28.	Remove gloves and all protective barriers and dispose of soiled supplies and equipment appropriately	❏	❏	_____
29.	Wash hands after patient contact and after removing gloves	❏	❏	_____
30.	Document and do patient teaching	❏	❏	_____
31.	Report any unexpected outcomes	❏	❏	_____

PERFORMANCE CHECKLIST 19-12

APPLYING A HOT, MOIST COMPRESS TO AN OPEN WOUND

		S	U	Comments
Prepare for procedure				
1.	Refer to medical record, care plan, or Kardex	❏	❏	_____
2.	Introduce self	❏	❏	_____
3.	Identify patient	❏	❏	_____
4.	Explain the procedure	❏	❏	_____
5.	Assess need for and provide patient teaching during procedure	❏	❏	_____
6.	Assess patient	❏	❏	_____
7.	Wash hands and don clean gloves	❏	❏	_____
8.	Assemble equipment and complete necessary charges	❏	❏	_____
9.	Prepare patient for intervention			
a.	Close door/pull privacy curtain	❏	❏	_____
b.	Raise bed to comfortable working height; lower side rail on side nearest the nurse	❏	❏	_____
c.	Position and drape patient as necessary	❏	❏	_____
During the skill:				
10.	Promote patient involvement as possible	❏	❏	_____
11.	Assess patient's tolerance	❏	❏	_____
12.	Describe sensations to be felt; explain precautions to prevent burning	❏	❏	_____
13.	Assess condition of exposed skin and wound on which compress is to be applied	❏	❏	_____
14.	Place waterproof pad under area to be treated	❏	❏	_____

	S	U	Comments
15. Assemble equipment; pour warmed solution into sterile container	❏	❏	_____
16. Open sterile packages and drop gauze into container to immerse in solution; set aquathermia pad (if used) to correct temperature and assess fluid level of unit	❏	❏	_____
17. Don disposable gloves; remove any existing dressings covering wound; dispose of gloves and dressings in proper receptacle	❏	❏	_____
18. Apply sterile gloves	❏	❏	_____
19. Apply sterile petroleum jelly (optional) with cotton swab to skin surrounding wound; do not apply jelly on impaired skin	❏	❏	_____
20. Pick up one layer of immersed gauze and squeeze out excess water	❏	❏	_____
21. Apply gauze lightly to open wound; observe response and ask whether patient feels discomfort; in a few seconds, lift edge of gauze to assess for erythema	❏	❏	_____
22. If patient tolerates compress, pack gauze snugly against wound; be certain all wound surfaces are covered by hot compress	❏	❏	_____
23. Wrap or cover moist compress with dry bath towel; if necessary, pin or tie in place	❏	❏	_____
24. Change hot compress frequently as ordered	❏	❏	_____
25. Apply aquathermia or waterproof heating pad over compress (optional); keep it in place for desired duration of application	❏	❏	_____
26. Assess patient periodically for discomfort or burning sensation; observe area of skin not covered by compress	❏	❏	_____
27. Remove pad, towel, and compress; again assess wound and condition of skin	❏	❏	_____
28. Apply dry, sterile dressing as ordered	❏	❏	_____

	S	**U**	**Comments**
29. Ask patient if any unusual burning sensation is noticed that was not felt before	❏	❏	_____

Postprocedure

30. Assist patient to a position of comfort and place needed items within easy reach; be certain patient has a means to call for assistance and knows how to use it	❏	❏	_____
31. Raise the side rails and lower the bed to the lowest position	❏	❏	_____
32. Remove gloves and all protective barriers; store or remove and dispose of soiled supplies and equipment appropriately	❏	❏	_____
33. Wash hands after patient contact and after removing gloves	❏	❏	_____
34. Document and do patient teaching	❏	❏	_____
35. Report an unexpected outcomes	❏	❏	_____

PERFORMANCE CHECKLIST 19-13

INITIATING INTRAVENOUS THERAPY

		S	U	Comments
Prepare for procedure				
1.	Refer to medical record, care plan, or Kardex	❏	❏	_____
2.	Introduce self	❏	❏	_____
3.	Identify patient	❏	❏	_____
4.	Explain the procedure and the reason it is to be done	❏	❏	_____
5.	Assess need for and provide patient teaching during procedure	❏	❏	_____
6.	Assess patient	❏	❏	_____
7.	Wash hands and don clean gloves	❏	❏	_____
8.	Assemble equipment and IV solution to be infused	❏	❏	_____
9.	Prepare patient for intervention			
	a. Close door/pull privacy curtain	❏	❏	_____
	b. Raise bed to comfortable working height; lower side rail on side nearest the nurse	❏	❏	_____
	c. Position and drape patient as necessary	❏	❏	_____
During the skill:				
10.	Promote patient involvement as possible	❏	❏	_____
11.	Assess patient's tolerance	❏	❏	_____
12.	Identify venipuncture sites	❏	❏	_____
13.	Apply tourniquet	❏	❏	_____
14.	Select venipuncture site	❏	❏	_____

	S	U	Comments
15. Cleanse site with alcohol swab, or other special agent such as Betadine, using friction	❏	❏	_____
16. Stretch skin taut and stabilize vein with nondominant hand	❏	❏	_____
17. Holding angiocatheter bevel up, pierce skin above and slightly to side of vein at 45-degree angle	❏	❏	_____
18. Lower angle to 10 degrees and enter vein wall; slight resistance and "pop" accompany entry into vein	❏	❏	_____
19. Follow vein lumen with tip of needle to ensure placement within vein, watching for blood return through angiocatheter backflow chamber	❏	❏	_____
20. Release tourniquet	❏	❏	_____
21. Holding guide needle in place, gently thread plastic catheter off needle and into vein	❏	❏	_____
22. Applying gentle pressure over catheter in vein, remove guide needle, and attach sterile connection end of primed tubing into catheter hub	❏	❏	_____
23. Stabilizing insertion site, slowly open flow valve to begin intravenous infusion	❏	❏	_____
24. Following agency policy, secure and dress site with tape, medications, and dressings	❏	❏	_____
25. Label site and tubing according to agency policy	❏	❏	_____
26. Adjust fluid flow rate according to accurate drop-rate calculations or set infusion rate on infusion pump	❏	❏	_____
27. If infusion pump is used, set milliliters to be infused (volume to be infused)	❏	❏	_____

Postprocedure

| 28. Assist patient to a position of comfort and place needed items within easy reach. Be certain patient has a means to call for assistance and knows how to use it | ❏ | ❏ | _____ |

	S	U	Comments
29. Raise the side rails and lower the bed to the lowest position	❏	❏	_____
30. Remove gloves and all protective barriers; store or remove and dispose of soiled supplies and equipment appropriately	❏	❏	_____
31. Wash hands after patient contact and after removing gloves	❏	❏	_____
32. Document and do patient teaching	❏	❏	_____
33. Report any unexpected outcomes	❏	❏	_____

PERFORMANCE CHECKLIST 19-14

Oxygen Administration

	S	U	Comments
Prepare for procedure			
1. Refer to medical record, care plan, or Kardex	❏	❏	_____
2. Introduce self	❏	❏	_____
3. Identify patient	❏	❏	_____
4. Explain the procedure and the reason it is to be done	❏	❏	_____
5. Assess need for (perform oximetry to obtain oxygen saturation) and provide patient teaching during procedure	❏	❏	_____
6. Assess patient	❏	❏	_____
7. Wash hands and don clean gloves	❏	❏	_____
8. Assemble equipment and complete necessary charges	❏	❏	_____
9. Prepare patient for intervention			
a. Close door/pull privacy curtain	❏	❏	_____
b. Raise bed to comfortable working height; lower side rail on side nearest the nurse	❏	❏	_____
c. Position and drape patient as necessary	❏	❏	_____
During the skill:			
10. Promote patient involvement as possible	❏	❏	_____
11. Assess patient's tolerance	❏	❏	_____
12. Explain necessary precautions during oxygen therapy	❏	❏	_____
13. Place patient in Fowler's or semi-Fowler's position	❏	❏	_____

		S	U	Comments
14.	Assess patient's airway	❏	❏	_____
15.	Consider laboratory reports	❏	❏	_____
16.	Suction any secretions obstructing the airway and reassess lung sounds with stethoscope	❏	❏	_____
17.	Fill humidifier container to designated level, if used: use sterile, distilled water or as prescribed	❏	❏	_____
18.	Attach flowmeter to humidifier and insert in proper oxygen source	❏	❏	_____
19.	Administer oxygen therapy	❏	❏	_____

Nasal cannula:

		S	U	Comments
a.	Attach nasal cannula to oxygen tubing, then attach to flowmeter	❏	❏	_____
b.	Place prongs in cup of water; adjust flow meter to 6–10 L to flush tubing and prongs with oxygen; wipe off water	❏	❏	_____
c.	Adjust flow rate to the prescribed amount	❏	❏	_____
d.	Place a nasal prong into each naris of the patient	❏	❏	_____
e.	Adjust liter flow per physician's order or to maintain oxygen saturation at 91% or greater	❏	❏	_____
f.	Adjust straps of the cannula over the ears and tighten under the chin	❏	❏	_____
g.	Place padding between strap and ears	❏	❏	_____
h.	Provide slack in tubing and secure to patient's garment	❏	❏	_____
i.	Maintain regular assessment			
(1)	Assess cannula frequently for possible obstruction	❏	❏	_____
(2)	Observe external nasal area, nares, and superior surface of both ears for skin impairment q6–8h	❏	❏	_____

		S	**U**	**Comments**

(3) Assess nares and prongs and cleanse with cotton-tipped applicator as needed; apply water-soluble lubricant to nares to prevent from drying ❏ ❏ _____

(4) Refer to physician's orders for any prescribed changes in flow rate ❏ ❏ _____

(5) Monitor oxygen saturation ❏ ❏ _____

(6) Maintain solution in humidifier container at appropriate level at all times ❏ ❏ _____

Nasal catheter:

j. Adjust flow rate to prescribed amount ❏ ❏ _____

k. Auscultate lung sounds ❏ ❏ _____

Face masks:

l. Adjust flow rate of oxygen per physician's order. Monitor oxygen saturation ❏ ❏ _____

m. Allow patient to hold mask and place your hand over patient's hand ❏ ❏ _____

n. Different types of masks may be used to meet patient's needs such as simple face mask, Venturi mask, partial rebreather mask, and nonrebreathing mask ❏ ❏ _____

o. Place mask over bridge of nose, then cover mouth ❏ ❏ _____

p. Adjust straps around patient's head and over ears; place cotton ball or gauze over ears under elastic straps ❏ ❏ _____

q. Observe reservoir bag if one is attached to mask ❏ ❏ _____

r. Maintain regular assessments:

(1) Remove mask and clean and dry skin regularly ❏ ❏ _____

		S	U	Comments
(2)	Refer to physician's orders for prescribed flow rate and any changes to maintain oxygen saturation of 91% or greater	❏	❏	_____
(3)	Maintain solution in humidifier container, if used, at appropriate level at all times	❏	❏	_____
s.	If face tent is used, a mist should always be present	❏	❏	_____

Postprocedure

		S	U	Comments
20.	Assist patient to a position of comfort and place needed items within easy reach; be certain patient has a means to call for assistance and knows how to use it	❏	❏	_____
21.	Raise the side rails and lower the bed to the lowest position	❏	❏	_____
22.	Remove gloves and all protective barriers and/or remove and dispose of soiled supplies and equipment appropriately	❏	❏	_____
23.	Wash hands after patient contact and after removing gloves	❏	❏	_____
24.	Document, including oxygen saturation levels, and do patient teaching	❏	❏	_____
25.	Report any unexpected outcomes	❏	❏	_____

PERFORMANCE CHECKLIST 19-15

TRACHEOSTOMY CARE AND SUCTIONING

		S	U	Comments
Prepare for procedure				
1.	Refer to medical record, care plan, or Kardex	❏	❏	_____
2.	Introduce self	❏	❏	_____
3.	Identify patient	❏	❏	_____
4.	Explain the procedure and the reason it is to be done	❏	❏	_____
5.	Assess need for and provide patient teaching during procedure	❏	❏	_____
6.	Assess patient	❏	❏	_____
7.	Wash hands and don clean gloves	❏	❏	_____
8.	Assemble equipment and complete necessary charges	❏	❏	_____
9.	Prepare patient for intervention			
a.	Close door/pull privacy curtain	❏	❏	_____
b.	Raise bed to comfortable working height; lower side rail on side nearest the nurse	❏	❏	_____
c.	Position and drape patient as necessary	❏	❏	_____
During the skill:				
10.	Promote patient involvement as possible	❏	❏	_____
11.	Assess patient's tolerance	❏	❏	_____
12.	Assess patient's tracheostomy	❏	❏	_____
13.	Position patient in semi-Fowler's position	❏	❏	_____
14.	Provide paper and pencil for patient	❏	❏	_____
15.	Position self at head of bed facing patient	❏	❏	_____

		S	U	Comments
16.	Auscultate lungs; monitor oxygen saturation	❏	❏	_____
17.	Place towel or prepackaged drape under tracheostomy and across chest	❏	❏	_____
18.	Prepare equipment and supplies on overbed table			
a.	Open suction catheter, leaving it in its wrapper, and attach it to suction machine	❏	❏	_____
b.	Pour cleansing solution (hydrogen peroxide) in one basin and rinsing solution (normal saline) in another basin	❏	❏	_____
c.	Turn on suction machine (120 mm Hg in adults); apply sterile glove; keep dominant hand sterile	❏	❏	_____
19.	Unlock and remove inner cannula; place in cleansing solution; place fingers on tabs of outer cannula	❏	❏	_____
20.	Suction inner aspect of outer cannula			
a.	Aspirate sterile rinsing solution through catheter	❏	❏	_____
b.	Ask patient to take several deep breaths or if patient is receiving oxygen, remove oxygen immediately before suctioning	❏	❏	_____
c.	Remove thumb from suction control or pinch catheter with gloved thumb and index finger; insert catheter 5–6 inches	❏	❏	_____
d.	Apply intermittent suction	❏	❏	_____
e.	Suction for a maximum of 10 seconds	❏	❏	_____
f.	Allow patient to rest between each episode of suctioning	❏	❏	_____
g.	Rinse catheter with sterile normal saline and repeat suctioning if needed	❏	❏	_____
h.	Turn off suction and dispose of catheter appropriately	❏	❏	_____

		S	U	Comments

21. Apply second sterile glove, if one-glove technique is used, or apply new pair of sterile gloves; clean inner cannula:

    a.   Use pipe cleaners and brush to clean inside and outside of inner cannula with hydrogen peroxide solution   ❏   ❏   _____

    b.   Place inner cannula in sterile normal saline solution, rinse thoroughly   ❏   ❏   _____

    c.   Inspect inner and outer areas of inner cannula; remove excess liquid   ❏   ❏   _____

    d.   Insert inner cannula and lock in place   ❏   ❏   _____

22. Clean skin around tracheostomy and tabs of outer cannula; use wipes that are free of lint around the tracheostomy opening   ❏   ❏   _____

23. Thoroughly rinse cleansing solution from skin; place dry, sterile dressing around tracheostomy face plate   ❏   ❏   _____

24. Change cotton tapes

    a.   Untie one side of cotton tape from outer cannula and replace with clean one   ❏   ❏   _____

    b.   Bring clean tape under back of neck   ❏   ❏   _____

    c.   Untie other side from outer cannula and replace with clean tape   ❏   ❏   _____

    d.   Tie ends of two clean cotton tapes together and position knot appropriately   ❏   ❏   _____

25. Auscultate lung sounds; monitor oxygen saturation   ❏   ❏   _____

26. Provide mouth care   ❏   ❏   _____

27. Remove gloves and all protective barriers and/or remove and dispose of soiled supplies and equipment appropriately   ❏   ❏   _____

28. Wash hands after patient contact and after removing gloves   ❏   ❏   _____

	S	U	Comments

Postprocedure

29. Assist patient to a position of comfort and place needed items within easy reach. Be certain patient has a means to call for assistance and knows how to use it ❑ ❑ _____

30. Raise the side rails and lower the bed to the lowest position ❑ ❑ _____

31. Place call light, paper, and pencil within easy reach ❑ ❑ _____

32. Reassess patient's tracheostomy ❑ ❑ _____

33. Document and do patient teaching ❑ ❑ _____

34. Report any unexpected outcomes ❑ ❑ _____

PERFORMANCE CHECKLIST 19-16

Care of the Patient with a Cuffed Tracheostomy Tube

	S	U	Comments

Prepare for procedure

		S	U	Comments
1.	Refer to medical record, care plan, or Kardex	❏	❏	_____
2.	Introduce self	❏	❏	_____
3.	Identify patient	❏	❏	_____
4.	Explain the procedure and the reason it is to be done	❏	❏	_____
5.	Assess need for and provide patient teaching during procedure	❏	❏	_____
6.	Assess patient	❏	❏	_____
7.	Wash hands and don clean gloves	❏	❏	_____
8.	Assemble equipment and complete necessary charges	❏	❏	_____
9.	Prepare patient for intervention			
a.	Close door/pull privacy curtain	❏	❏	_____
b.	Raise bed to comfortable working height; lower side rail on side nearest the nurse	❏	❏	_____
c.	Position and drape patient as necessary	❏	❏	_____

During the skill:

		S	U	Comments
10.	Promote patient involvement as possible	❏	❏	_____
11.	Assess patient's tolerance; monitor oxygen saturation	❏	❏	_____
12.	Suction patient as in skill 19-15 steps 12 through 20h; connect syringe to pilot balloon valve	❏	❏	_____
13.	Position stethoscope in sternal notch or above tracheostomy tube and listen for minimal amount of air leak at end of inspiration	❏	❏	_____

	S	U	Comments
14. Remove all air from cuff if no air leak is auscultated	❏	❏	_____
15. While listening with stethoscope, slowly inflate cuff with 0.5–1 ml of air at a time; when no air leak is heard, stop injecting air and slowly withdraw up to 0.5 ml of air until air leak is auscultated with stethoscope	❏	❏	_____
16. If excessive air leak is heard, slowly add air as in step 15	❏	❏	_____
17. Remove stethoscope and cleanse diaphragm with alcohol swab	❏	❏	_____
18. Do not leave syringe attached to pilot balloon valve; remove syringe and either discard in proper container or store per agency's policy	❏	❏	_____

Postprocedure

	S	U	Comments
19. Assist patient to a position of comfort and place needed items within easy reach; be certain patient has a means to call for assistance and knows how to use it	❏	❏	_____
20. Raise the side rails and lower the bed to the lowest position	❏	❏	_____
21. Remove gloves and all protective barriers and/or remove and dispose of soiled supplies and equipment appropriately	❏	❏	_____
22. Wash hands after patient contact and after removing gloves	❏	❏	_____
23. Document and do patient teaching	❏	❏	_____
24. Report any unexpected outcomes	❏	❏	_____

PERFORMANCE CHECKLIST 19-17

CLEARING THE AIRWAY

	S	U	Comments
Prepare for procedure			
1. Refer to medical record, care plan, or Kardex	❏	❏	_____
2. Introduce self	❏	❏	_____
3. Identify patient	❏	❏	_____
4. Explain the procedure and the reason it is to be done	❏	❏	_____
5. Assess need for and provide patient teaching during procedure	❏	❏	_____
6. Assess patient	❏	❏	_____
7. Wash hands and don clean gloves	❏	❏	_____
8. Assemble equipment and complete necessary charges	❏	❏	_____
9. Prepare patient for intervention			
a. Close door/pull privacy curtain	❏	❏	_____
b. Raise bed to comfortable working height; lower side rail on side nearest the nurse	❏	❏	_____
c. Position and drape patient as necessary	❏	❏	_____
During the skill:			
10. Promote patient involvement as possible	❏	❏	_____
11. Assess patient's tolerance; monitor oxygen saturation	❏	❏	_____
12. Position patient			
a. If patient is alert and conscious, place in semi-Fowler's position with head to one side	❏	❏	_____

		S	U	Comments
b.	If patient is unconscious, place in side-lying position facing nurse	❑	❑	_____
	(1) Place towel lengthwise under patient's chin and over pillow	❑	❑	_____
13.	Pour sterile normal saline solution into sterile container	❑	❑	_____
14.	Turn on suction machine, and select appropriate suction pressure, usually 120 mm Hg for adults	❑	❑	_____
15.	Select appropriate catheter size	❑	❑	_____
16.	Aspirate solution through catheter	❑	❑	_____
17.	Remove thumb from Y-connector opening or pinch catheter with thumb and index finger; if using suction catheter with vent, remove thumb from vent opening	❑	❑	_____
18.	Insert catheter	❑	❑	_____

Oropharyngeal suctioning

		S	U	Comments
a.	Gently insert Yankauer into one side of mouth	❑	❑	_____
b.	Glide Yankauer toward oropharynx without suction	❑	❑	_____
c.	Apply suction and move Yankauer tonsillar tip catheter around mouth until secretions are cleared	❑	❑	_____
d.	Encourage patient to cough	❑	❑	_____
e.	Rinse Yankauer; turn off suction	❑	❑	_____
f.	Repeat procedure as necessary	❑	❑	_____

Nasopharyngeal suctioning

		S	U	Comments
g.	Holding catheter, assess for correct length of insertion	❑	❑	_____
h.	Lubricate catheter with water-soluble lubricant	❑	❑	_____

		S	U	Comments
i.	Hold catheter to observe its natural curvature and gently insert catheter into one side of nasal passage	❏	❏	_____

Nasotracheal suctioning

		S	U	Comments
j.	Holding catheter, measure for correct length	❏	❏	_____
k.	Lubricate catheter with water-soluble lubricant	❏	❏	_____
l.	Ask patient if either side of nose is obstructed; use unobstructed side; hold catheter to observe its natural curvature and gently insert catheter into one side of nasal passage	❏	❏	_____
m.	Stimulate coughing reflex, or ask patient to cough to guide catheter into trachea; if no cough reflex is present or if patient cannot assist, insert catheter when patient inhales	❏	❏	_____
19.	Apply intermittent suction	❏	❏	_____
20.	Observe patient closely and limit suction for the appropriate time	❏	❏	_____
21.	Repeat suctioning if needed	❏	❏	_____
22.	Allow 1–2 minutes rest between suctioning if procedure must be repeated; if oxygen is administered by nasal cannula, mask, or other means, reapply oxygen during rest period	❏	❏	_____
23.	If patient is alert and can cooperate, request patient to breathe deeply and cough	❏	❏	_____
24.	When suctioning is complete, suction between cheeks and gum line and under tongue; suction mouth last	❏	❏	_____
25.	Place catheter in solution and supply suction	❏	❏	_____
26.	Discard catheter	❏	❏	_____
27.	Place sterile, unopened catheter at patient's bedside	❏	❏	_____

		S	U	Comments
28.	Provide mouth care	❏	❏	_____
29.	Assess patient's breathing patterns	❏	❏	_____
30.	Monitor oxygen saturation	❏	❏	_____

Postprocedure

31.	Assist patient to a position of comfort and place needed items within easy reach. Be certain patient has a means to call for assistance and knows how to use it	❏	❏	_____
32.	Raise the side rails and lower the bed to the lowest position	❏	❏	_____
33.	Remove gloves and all protective barriers and/or remove and dispose of soiled supplies and equipment appropriately	❏	❏	_____
34.	Wash hands	❏	❏	_____
35.	Document and do patient teaching	❏	❏	_____
36.	Report any unexpected outcomes	❏	❏	_____

PERFORMANCE CHECKLIST 19-18

CATHETERIZATION: MALE AND FEMALE

	S	U	Comments
Prepare for procedure			
1. Refer to medical record, care plan, or Kardex	❏	❏	_____
2. Introduce self	❏	❏	_____
3. Identify patient	❏	❏	_____
4. Explain the procedure and the reason it is to be done	❏	❏	_____
5. Assess need for and provide patient teaching during procedure	❏	❏	_____
6. Assess patient	❏	❏	_____
7. Wash hands and don clean gloves	❏	❏	_____
8. Assemble equipment and complete necessary charges	❏	❏	_____
9. Prepare patient for intervention			
a. Close door/pull privacy curtain	❏	❏	_____
b. Raise bed to comfortable working height; lower side rail on side nearest the nurse	❏	❏	_____
c. Position and drape patient as necessary	❏	❏	_____
During the skill:			
10. Promote patient involvement as possible	❏	❏	_____
11. Assess patient's tolerance	❏	❏	_____
12. Arrange for extra nursing personnel to assist	❏	❏	_____
13. Position patient	❏	❏	_____
a. Male: Supine position with thighs slightly abducted	❏	❏	_____
b. Female: Dorsal recumbent position with knees flexed, soles of feet flat on bed, and feet about 2 feet apart	❏	❏	_____

	S	U	Comments
14. Drape patient with bath blanket	❏	❏	_____
15. Place waterproof, absorbent pad under patient's buttocks	❏	❏	_____
16. Arrange supplies and equipment on bedside table; provide a good light	❏	❏	_____
17. Don clean gloves and wash perineal area	❏	❏	_____
18. Remove disposable gloves and place in proper receptacle	❏	❏	_____
19. Facing patient, stand on left side of bed if right-handed (on right side if left-handed)	❏	❏	_____
20. Open packaging using sterile technique; don sterile gloves	❏	❏	_____
21. If indwelling catheter is used, test balloon appropriately	❏	❏	_____
22. Add antiseptic to cotton balls; open lubricant container; lubricate catheter the appropriate length	❏	❏	_____
23. Wrap edges of sterile drape around gloved hands and request patient to raise hips, then slide drape under patient's buttocks	❏	❏	_____
24. Cleanse perineal area using forceps to hold cotton balls soaked in antiseptic solution			
a. Male: If male is not circumcised, retract foreskin with nondominant hand; if erection does occur, discontinue procedure momentarily			
(1) Grasp penis at shaft below glans with one hand; continue to hold throughout insertion of catheter	❏	❏	_____
(2) With other hand, use forceps to hold cotton balls soaked in antiseptic solution	❏	❏	_____
(3) Cleanse meatus in circular motion	❏	❏	_____
(4) Repeat cleansing two more times using sterile cotton balls each time	❏	❏	_____

	S	**U**	**Comments**

b. Female

    (1) Have assistant hold pen light or flashlight to provide adequate lighting   ❏   ❏ _____

    (2) Spread labia minora with thumb and index finger of nondominant hand and be prepared to hold throughout the insertion of the catheter   ❏   ❏ _____

    (3) With other hand, use forceps to hold cotton balls soaked in antiseptic solution   ❏   ❏ _____

    (4) Cleanse area from clitoris toward anus, using a different sterile cotton ball each time—first to the right of the meatus, then to the left of the meatus, then down the center over meatus   ❏   ❏ _____

25. Pick up catheter with free sterile, gloved hand near the tip; hold remaining part of catheter coiled in hands; place distal end in basin   ❏   ❏ _____

26. Insert catheter gently, 15–18 cm (6–7 inches) for male or 5–10 cm (2–4 inches) for female   ❏   ❏ _____

27. Collect urine specimen, if needed   ❏   ❏ _____

28. Type of catheter

    a. Indwelling catheter

      (1) Inflate balloon with required amount of normal saline or sterile water   ❏   ❏ _____

      (2) Pull gently to feel resistance   ❏   ❏ _____

      (3) Attach drainage bag below the level of bladder (most catheters are presealed to the collecting tube of the drainage system)   ❏   ❏ _____

      (4) Attach collection bag to side of bed   ❏   ❏ _____

      (5) Secure catheter to patient

        • Male: Tape catheter to top of thigh appropriately   ❏   ❏ _____

	S	U	Comments
• Female: Tape catheter to inner thigh appropriately	❏	❏	_____
(6) Clip drainage tubing to bed linen appropriately	❏	❏	_____
b. Straight catheter			
(1) Hold coiled catheter in hand with opening draining into sterile basin or into presealed plastic drainage bag	❏	❏	_____
(2) Empty bladder	❏	❏	_____
(3) Withdraw catheter slowly	❏	❏	_____
29. Dry perineal area	❏	❏	_____

Postprocedure

	S	U	Comments
30. Assist patient to a position of comfort and place needed items within easy reach; be certain patient has a means to call for assistance and knows how to use it	❏	❏	_____
31. Raise the side rails and lower the bed to the lowest position	❏	❏	_____
32. Assess flow of urine and drainage tubing setup	❏	❏	_____
33. Remove gloves and all protective barriers and/or remove and dispose of soiled supplies and equipment appropriately	❏	❏	_____
34. Wash hands after patient contact and after removing gloves	❏	❏	_____
35. Document type of catheter used, amount and color of urine and do patient teaching	❏	❏	_____
36. Report any unexpected outcomes	❏	❏	_____
37. Label urine specimen appropriately	❏	❏	_____
38. Transport to laboratory immediately	❏	❏	_____

PERFORMANCE CHECKLIST 19-19

PERFORMING ROUTINE CATHETER CARE

	S	U	Comments

Prepare for procedure

1. Refer to medical record, care plan, or Kardex ❏ ❏ _____

2. Introduce self ❏ ❏ _____

3. Identify patient ❏ ❏ _____

4. Explain the procedure and the reason it is to be done ❏ ❏ _____

5. Assess need for and provide patient teaching during procedure ❏ ❏ _____

6. Assess patient ❏ ❏ _____

7. Wash hands and don clean gloves ❏ ❏ _____

8. Assemble equipment and complete necessary charges ❏ ❏ _____

9. Prepare patient for intervention

   a. Close door/pull privacy curtain ❏ ❏ _____

   b. Raise bed to comfortable working height; lower side rail on side nearest the nurse ❏ ❏ _____

   c. Position and drape patient as necessary ❏ ❏ _____

During the skill:

10. Promote patient involvement as possible ❏ ❏ _____

11. Assess patient's tolerance ❏ ❏ _____

12. Position patient

    a. Male: In bed in supine position ❏ ❏ _____

    b. Female: In bed in dorsal recumbent position ❏ ❏ _____

	S	U	Comments
13. Place waterproof disposable pad under patient's buttocks and to the side from which catheter care will be given	❏	❏	_____
14. Drape patient with bath blanket, exposing only perineal area	❏	❏	_____
15. If using sterile catheter care kit:			
a. Open supplies using sterile technique and arrange on bedside table	❏	❏	_____
b. Don sterile gloves	❏	❏	_____
c. Place cotton balls in sterile basin and saturate with sterile solution	❏	❏	_____
d. With one hand expose urethral meatus:			
(1) Male: retract foreskin, then hold penis erect	❏	❏	_____
(2) Female: gently retract labia minora away from urinary meatus and hold in position	❏	❏	_____
e. Wash the area at the meatus and around the catheter with cotton balls saturated with sterile solution			
(1) Male			
• With one cotton ball, cleanse around meatus and catheter in a circular motion	❏	❏	_____
• Repeat twice more, using different cotton balls each time	❏	❏	_____
(2) Female			
• With one cotton ball, swab to one side of labia minora from anterior to posterior	❏	❏	_____
• Repeat with second cotton ball on opposite side	❏	❏	_____

	S	U	Comments

- Repeat with third cotton ball down middle over meatus and around catheter ❏ ❏ _____

f. Discard soiled cotton balls in other basin in kit ❏ ❏ _____

g. With forceps, pick up cotton ball soaked in antiseptic solution or mild soap and water and cleanse around catheter from urethral opening ❏ ❏ _____

16. If using a collection of sterile supplies:

a. Open separate sterile packages observing sterile technique ❏ ❏ _____

b. Don clean gloves ❏ ❏ _____

c. Arrange refuse bag ❏ ❏ _____

d. Cleanse the perineal area with mild soap and warm water; pat dry

(1) Male: retract foreskin then hold the penis erect ❏ ❏ _____

(2) Female: gently retract labia away from urinary meatus and hold in position ❏ ❏ _____

e. Apply in appropriate amount of sterile anti-infective ointment (if used) on sterile cotton-tipped applicator and gently apply around catheter at site of insertion (this is seldom used now) ❏ ❏ _____

f. Release labia of female patient; replace foreskin of male patient ❏ ❏ _____

17. Retape catheter to thigh ❏ ❏ _____

18. Observe meatus, catheter, and surrounding tissue to assess normal or abnormal condition; determine presence or absence of inflammation, edema, malodorous exudate, color of tissue, and burning sensation ❏ ❏ _____

	S	U	Comments

Postprocedure

19. Assist patient to a position of comfort and place needed items within easy reach; be certain patient has a means to call for assistance and knows how to use it ❑ ❑ _____

20. Raise the side rails and lower the bed to the lowest position ❑ ❑ _____

21. Remove gloves and all protective barriers and/or remove and dispose of soiled supplies and equipment appropriately ❑ ❑ _____

22. Wash hands after patient contact and after removing gloves ❑ ❑ _____

23. Document and do patient teaching ❑ ❑ _____

24. Report any unexpected outcomes ❑ ❑ _____

PERFORMANCE CHECKLIST 19-20

CATHETER IRRIGATION: OPEN, INTERMITTENT, CONTINUOUS, AND BLADDER INSTILLATION

	S	U	Comments
Prepare for procedure			
1. Refer to medical record, care plan, or Kardex	❏	❏	_____
2. Introduce self	❏	❏	_____
3. Identify patient	❏	❏	_____
4. Explain the procedure and the reason it is to be done	❏	❏	_____
5. Assess need for and provide patient teaching	❏	❏	_____
6. Assess patient	❏	❏	_____
7. Wash hands and don clean gloves	❏	❏	_____
8. Assemble equipment and complete necessary charges	❏	❏	_____
9. Prepare patient for intervention			
a. Close door/pull privacy curtain	❏	❏	_____
b. Raise bed to comfortable working height; lower side rail on side nearest the nurse	❏	❏	_____
c. Position and drape patient as necessary	❏	❏	_____
During the skill:			
10. Promote patient involvement as possible	❏	❏	_____
11. Assess patient	❏	❏	_____
12. Place waterproof absorbent pad under patient's buttocks and to the side from which bladder irrigation will be done	❏	❏	_____
13. Arrange supplies and equipment at bedside on overbed table	❏	❏	_____

		S	U	Comments
14.	Open method			
	a. Pour sterile irrigating solution (normal saline unless otherwise specified) into sterile graduated container and recap solution bottle; irrigating solution should be at room temperature	❑	❑	_____
	b. Don sterile gloves	❑	❑	_____
	c. Place sterile basin between patient's legs, close to perineal area	❑	❑	_____
	d. Disconnect catheter from drainage system and plug drainage tubing with sterile plug	❑	❑	_____
	e. Draw 30 ml of sterile solution into syringe	❑	❑	_____
	f. Cleanse catheter end with antiseptic swab	❑	❑	_____
	g. Place tip of syringe into end of catheter and gently insert solution	❑	❑	_____
	h. Withdraw syringe and allow solution to drain into basin by gravity	❑	❑	_____
	i. If solution does not return, turn patient on side facing nurse	❑	❑	_____
	j. Repeat injection of solution until amount ordered is injected and returned	❑	❑	_____
	k. Remove plug from drainage tubing, and connect tubing to catheter	❑	❑	_____
	l. Measure solution (to determine amount returned and amount of urine expelled)	❑	❑	_____
15.	Closed intermittent method (repeat steps 1 to 13)			
	a. Pour sterile irrigating solution (normal saline unless otherwise specified) into graduated container	❑	❑	_____
	b. Draw up sterile solution into syringe	❑	❑	_____
	c. Clamp catheter below injection port	❑	❑	_____
	d. Cleanse port with antiseptic	❑	❑	_____

		S	**U**	**Comments**
e.	Insert needle of syringe into port	❏	❏	_____
f.	Inject solution into catheter slowly	❏	❏	_____

16. Closed continuous method or continuous bladder irrigation (CBI)

		S	**U**	**Comments**
a.	Set up irrigating solution (normal saline unless otherwise specified) by attaching tubing to irrigation bag	❏	❏	_____
b.	Clamp off tubing so no solution flows through	❏	❏	_____
c.	Suspend bag on IV pole	❏	❏	_____
d.	Open clamp and allow solution to flow through tubing	❏	❏	_____
e.	Cleanse irrigating lumen on end of triple lumen catheter	❏	❏	_____
f.	Connect irrigating solution tubing to catheter lumen	❏	❏	_____
g.	Restore flow as ordered; run drip rate to keep drainage system clear	❏	❏	_____

17. Bladder instillation

		S	**U**	**Comments**
a.	Disconnect catheter from tubing—stabilize tubing to prevent touching the floor (triple lumen catheter does not require disconnection from drainage tubing)	❏	❏	_____
b.	Cleanse end of catheter with antiseptic swab	❏	❏	_____
c.	Draw medication or solution ordered into syringe	❏	❏	_____
d.	Place tip of syringe into end of catheter and slowly inject medication or solution ordered	❏	❏	_____
e.	Clamp off end of catheter for period of time necessary; then reconnect catheter and tubing, making certain the system is tightly connected	❏	❏	_____

		S	U	Comments
f.	Measure solution	❏	❏	_____

Postprocedure

18. Assist patient to a position of comfort and place needed items within easy reach; be certain patient has a means to call for assistance and knows how to use it ❏ ❏ _____

19. Raise the side rails and lower the bed to the lowest position ❏ ❏ _____

20. Remove gloves and all protective barriers and/or remove and dispose of soiled supplies and equipment appropriately ❏ ❏ _____

21. Wash hands after patient contact and after removing gloves ❏ ❏ _____

22. Document and do patient teaching ❏ ❏ _____

23. Report any unexpected outcomes ❏ ❏ _____

PERFORMANCE CHECKLIST 19-21

PERFORMING A VAGINAL IRRIGATION/DOUCHE

		S	U	Comments

Prepare for procedure

		S	U	Comments
1.	Refer to medical record, care plan, or Kardex	❏	❏	_____
2.	Introduce self	❏	❏	_____
3.	Identify patient	❏	❏	_____
4.	Explain the procedure and the reason it is to be done	❏	❏	_____
5.	Assess need for and provide patient teaching during procedure	❏	❏	_____
6.	Assess patient	❏	❏	_____
7.	Wash hands and don clean gloves	❏	❏	_____
8.	Assemble equipment and complete necessary charges	❏	❏	_____
9.	Prepare patient for intervention			
	a. Close door/pull privacy curtain	❏	❏	_____
	b. Raise bed to comfortable working height; lower side rail on side nearest the nurse	❏	❏	_____
	c. Position and drape patient as necessary	❏	❏	_____

During the skill:

		S	U	Comments
10.	Promote patient involvement as possible	❏	❏	_____
11.	Assess patient's tolerance	❏	❏	_____
12.	Prepare equipment			
	a. Solution should be at body temperature	❏	❏	_____
	b. Allow some solution to drain down the tubing out through the nozzle into bedpan	❏	❏	_____

		S	U	Comments
13.	Gently retract labial folds and direct nozzle toward the sacrum, following the floor of the vagina	❏	❏	_____
14.	Raise the container approximately 30–50 cm (12–20 in) above level of vagina	❏	❏	_____
15.	Insert nozzle appropriately	❏	❏	_____
16.	Allow solution to flow while inserting and rotating nozzle	❏	❏	_____
17.	Instruct patient to tighten perineal muscles as if to suppress urination and then relax; repeat four to five times during procedure	❏	❏	_____
18.	Administer all of the solution while rotating nozzle gently during instillation	❏	❏	_____
19.	Withdraw nozzle and assist patient to a comfortable position while she remains on the bedpan	❏	❏	_____
20.	Allow patient to remain on bedpan a short time (10 minutes), then don clean gloves; remove bedpan, assessing results; dispose of remaining solution in proper manner	❏	❏	_____
21.	Cleanse and dry patient or allow her to cleanse and dry herself	❏	❏	_____

Postprocedure

		S	U	Comments
22.	Assist patient to a position of comfort and place needed items within easy reach. Be certain patient has a means to call for assistance and knows how to use it	❏	❏	_____
23.	Raise the side rails and lower the bed to the lowest position	❏	❏	_____
24.	Remove gloves and all protective barriers and/or remove and dispose of soiled supplies and equipment appropriately	❏	❏	_____
25.	Wash hands after patient contact and after removing gloves	❏	❏	_____
26.	Document and do patient teaching	❏	❏	_____
27.	Report any unexpected outcomes	❏	❏	_____

PERFORMANCE CHECKLIST 19-22

INSERTING A NASOGASTRIC TUBE

	S	U	Comments
Prepare for procedure			
1. Refer to medical record, care plan, or Kardex	❏	❏	_____
2. Introduce self	❏	❏	_____
3. Identify patient	❏	❏	_____
4. Explain the procedure and the reason it is to be done	❏	❏	_____
5. Assess need for and provide patient teaching during procedure	❏	❏	_____
6. Assess patient	❏	❏	_____
7. Wash hands and don clean gloves	❏	❏	_____
8. Assemble equipment and complete necessary charges	❏	❏	_____
9. Prepare patient for intervention			
a. Close door/pull privacy curtain	❏	❏	_____
b. Raise bed to comfortable working height; lower side rail on side nearest the nurse	❏	❏	_____
c. Position and drape patient as necessary	❏	❏	_____
During the skill:			
10. Promote patient involvement as possible	❏	❏	_____
11. Assess patient's tolerance	❏	❏	_____
12. Assess patient for condition of nares and oral cavity	❏	❏	_____
13. Palpate patient's abdomen	❏	❏	_____
14. Position patient in high Fowler's position with pillow behind head and shoulders	❏	❏	_____

	S	U	Comments
15. Stand at right side of bed if right-handed and left side if left-handed	❏	❏	_____
16. Place bath towel over patient's chest; give tissues to patient	❏	❏	_____
17. Instruct patient to relax and breathe normally while occluding one naris; repeat this action for other naris	❏	❏	_____
18. Measure distance to insert tube correctly (measure distance from tip of nose to earlobe to xiphoid process of sternum)	❏	❏	_____
19. Mark length of tube to be inserted with piece of tape or note distance from next tube marking	❏	❏	_____
20. Curve end of tube tightly around index finger; release	❏	❏	_____
21. Lubricate end of tube generously with water-soluble lubricating jelly	❏	❏	_____
22. Initially instruct patient to extend neck back against pillow; insert tube slowly through naris with curved end pointing downward	❏	❏	_____
23. Continue to pass tube along floor of nasal passage, aiming down toward ear; when resistance is felt, apply gentle downward pressure to advance tube (do not force past resistance)	❏	❏	_____
24. If resistance continues, withdraw tube, allow patient to rest, relubricate tube, and insert into other naris	❏	❏	_____
25. Continue insertion of tube until just past nasopharynx by gently rotating tube toward opposite naris			
a. Stop tube advancement, allow patient to relax, and provide tissues	❏	❏	_____
b. Explain that the next step requires swallowing	❏	❏	_____

	S	U	Comments

26. With tube just above oropharynx, instruct patient to flex head forward and dry swallow or suck in air through straw; advance with each swallow; if patient has trouble swallowing and is allowed fluids, offer glass of water; advance tube with each swallow of water; while advancing the tube in an unconscious patient (or in a patient who cannot swallow), stroke the patient's neck ❏ ❏ _____

27. If patient begins to cough, gag, or choke, stop tube advancement; instruct patient to breathe easily and take sips of water ❏ ❏ _____

28. If patient continues to cough, pull tube back slightly ❏ ❏ _____

29. If patient continues to gag, assess back of oral pharynx using flashlight and tongue blade ❏ ❏ _____

30. After patient relaxes, continue to advance tube desired distance ❏ ❏ _____

31. Ask patient to talk ❏ ❏ _____

32. Assess posterior pharynx for presence of coiled tube ❏ ❏ _____

33. Attach cone-tipped syringe to end of tube; aspirate gently back on syringe to obtain gastric contents ❏ ❏ _____

34. Measure pH of aspirate with color-coded pH paper ❏ ❏ _____

35. If tube is not in the stomach, advance another 2.5–5 cm (1–2 in) and repeat step 33 ❏ ❏ _____

36. After tube is properly inserted, clamp end or connect it to suction ❏ ❏ _____

37. Cleanse nose with alcohol and Skin Prep for better adherence of nasal guard ❏ ❏ _____

38. Secure tube to nose with a nasal guard; avoid putting pressure on nares ❏ ❏ _____

39. Clean the skin over the nose with alcohol to remove any skin oils or soil and coat with Skin Prep before applying the nose guard ❏ ❏ _____

	S	U	Comments
40. Fasten end of tube to gown by looping rubber band around tube in slip knot; pin rubber band to gown	❑	❑	_____
41. Unless physician orders otherwise, head of bed should be elevated 30 degrees	❑	❑	_____

Postprocedure

	S	U	Comments
42. Assist patient to a position of comfort and place needed items within easy reach; be certain patient has a means to call for assistance and knows how to use it	❑	❑	_____
43. Raise the side rails and lower the bed to the lowest position	❑	❑	_____
44. Remove gloves and all protective barriers and/or remove and dispose of soiled supplies and equipment	❑	❑	_____
45. Wash hands after patient contact and after removing gloves	❑	❑	_____
46. Document and do patient teaching	❑	❑	_____
47. Report any unexpected outcomes	❑	❑	_____

PERFORMANCE CHECKLIST 19-23

NASOGASTRIC TUBE IRRIGATION

		S	U	Comments
Prepare for procedure				
1.	Refer to medical record, care plan, or Kardex	❏	❏	_____
2.	Introduce self	❏	❏	_____
3.	Identify patient	❏	❏	_____
4.	Explain the procedure and the reason it is to be done	❏	❏	_____
5.	Assess need for and provide patient teaching during procedure			
6.	Assess patient	❏	❏	_____
7.	Wash hands and don clean gloves	❏	❏	_____
8.	Assemble equipment and complete necessary charges	❏	❏	_____
9.	Prepare patient for intervention			
a.	Close door/pull privacy curtain	❏	❏	_____
b.	Raise bed to comfortable working height; lower side rail on side nearest the nurse	❏	❏	_____
c.	Position and drape patient as necessary	❏	❏	_____
During the skill:				
10.	Promote patient involvement as possible	❏	❏	_____
11.	Assess patient's tolerance	❏	❏	_____
13.	Place patient in semi-Fowler's position	❏	❏	_____
14.	Verify that tube is in right place by attaching syringe to end of tube and aspirating for stomach content	❏	❏	_____
15.	Assess abdomen	❏	❏	_____

	S	U	Comments
16. Pour normal saline into container; draw up 30 ml (or amount ordered) into piston syringe	❏	❏	_____
17. Clamp connection tubing distal to connection site for drainage or suction apparatus; disconnect tubing and lay end on a towel or waterproof pad	❏	❏	_____
18. Insert tip of irrigating syringe into end of NG tube; hold syringe with tip pointed toward the floor and instill 30 ml or ordered amount saline slowly and evenly (**do not force solution**)	❏	❏	_____
19. If resistance is met, assess tubing for kinks, change patient's position, and repeat attempt; if resistance continues, confer with RN or physician	❏	❏	_____
20. Withdraw fluid into syringe and measure; continue irrigating with ordered amount of saline until purpose of irrigation has been accomplished	❏	❏	_____
21. Reconnect NG tube to suction, introduce 30 ml of air into blue air vent lumen to clear air vent tubing; do not put liquid irrigant into blue airway lumen; secure airway lumen above level of stomach	❏	❏	_____
22. Note amount of saline instilled and withdrawn; subtract amount instilled from amount withdrawn and record difference as output	❏	❏	_____

Postprocedure

	S	U	Comments
23. Assist patient to a position of comfort and place needed items within easy reach; be certain patient has a means to call for assistance and knows how to use it	❏	❏	_____
24. Raise the side rails and lower the bed to the lowest position	❏	❏	_____
25. Remove gloves and all protective barriers and/or remove and dispose of soiled supplies and equipment appropriately	❏	❏	_____
26. Wash hands after patient contact and after removing gloves	❏	❏	_____
27. Document and do patient teaching	❏	❏	_____
28. Report any unexpected outcomes	❏	❏	_____

PERFORMANCE CHECKLIST 19-24

GASTRIC AND INTESTINAL SUCTIONING CARE

	S	**U**	**Comments**
Prepare for procedure			
1. Refer to medical record, care plan, or Kardex	❑	❑	_____
2. Introduce self	❑	❑	_____
3. Identify patient	❑	❑	_____
4. Explain the procedure and the reason it is to be done	❑	❑	_____
5. Assess need for and provide patient teaching during procedure	❑	❑	_____
6. Assess patient	❑	❑	_____
7. Wash hands and don clean gloves	❑	❑	_____
8. Assemble equipment and complete necessary charges	❑	❑	_____
9. Prepare patient for intervention			
a. Close door/pull privacy curtain	❑	❑	_____
b. Raise bed to comfortable working height; lower side rail on side nearest the nurse	❑	❑	_____
c. Position and drape patient as necessary	❑	❑	_____
During the skill:			
10. Promote patient involvement as possible	❑	❑	_____
11. Assess patient's tolerance	❑	❑	_____
12. Assess suction apparatus	❑	❑	_____
13. For wall suction:			
a. Make certain pressure gauge connections are tight	❑	❑	_____

		S	U	Comments
b.	Make certain pressure indicated on gauge is as ordered or according to agency policy; 80–100 mm Hg pressure above 120 mm Hg results in gastric bleeding	❑	❑	_____
c.	Suction is set on intermittent or continuous as ordered	❑	❑	_____

14. Assess patient:

		S	U	Comments
a.	Oral/nasal cavities	❑	❑	_____
b.	Abdomen for bowel sounds and extent of distention (be certain to turn off wall suctioning during assessment to prevent hearing Salem sump sounds)	❑	❑	_____
c.	NPO status	❑	❑	_____
d.	Lips and oral mucosa	❑	❑	_____

		S	U	Comments
15.	Ensure that tubing is not kinked and that patient is not lying on tubing	❑	❑	_____
16.	Pin NG tube to patient's gown with enough slack to allow movement	❑	❑	_____
17.	Verify that drainage is moving through tubing to drainage collection bottle	❑	❑	_____
18.	For Salem sump tube see that vent is pointing upward; listen at opening of blue air vent; if no hissing sounds are heard, instruct patient to cough or reposition to the right or left Sims' or supine position; it may be necessary to momentarily disconnect the NG tube from the suction tubing; be certain to reconnect immediately	❑	❑	_____
19.	Measure amount of drainage in bottle, noting color; empty when becoming full and at end of each shift	❑	❑	_____

Postprocedure

		S	U	Comments
20.	Assist patient to a position of comfort and place needed items within easy reach; be certain patient has a means to call for assistance and knows how to use it	❑	❑	_____

Student Name _____ Date _____ Instructor's Name _____

	S	U	Comments
21. Raise the side rails and lower the bed to the lowest position	❏	❏	_____
22. Remove gloves and all protective barriers and/or remove and dispose of soiled supplies and equipment appropriately	❏	❏	_____
23. Wash hands after patient contact and after removing gloves	❏	❏	_____
24. Document and do patient teaching	❏	❏	_____
25. Report any unexpected outcomes	❏	❏	_____

PERFORMANCE CHECKLIST 19-25

NASOGASTRIC TUBE REMOVAL

		S	U	Comments

Prepare for procedure

1. Refer to medical record, care plan, or Kardex ❏ ❏ _____

2. Introduce self ❏ ❏ _____

3. Identify patient ❏ ❏ _____

4. Explain the procedure and the reason it is to be done ❏ ❏ _____

5. Assess need for and provide patient teaching during procedure ❏ ❏ _____

6. Assess patient ❏ ❏ _____

7. Wash hands and don clean gloves ❏ ❏ _____

8. Assemble equipment and complete necessary charges ❏ ❏ _____

9. Prepare patient for intervention

   a. Close door/pull privacy curtain ❏ ❏ _____

   b. Raise bed to comfortable working height; lower side rail on side nearest the nurse ❏ ❏ _____

   c. Position and drape patient as necessary ❏ ❏ _____

During the skill:

10. Promote patient involvement as possible ❏ ❏ _____

11. Assess patient's tolerance ❏ ❏ _____

12. Reassure that removal is less distressing than insertion ❏ ❏ _____

13. Assess:

   a. Patient's abdomen for bowel sounds (turn off wall suction during assessment to prevent misinterpreting Salem sump sounds for peristalsis) ❏ ❏ _____

	S	U	Comments
b. Patient's nasal and oral cavity	❏	❏	_____
14. If tube is attached to suction, turn off suction machine and disconnect tubing, remove nose guard, and unfasten pin from gown	❏	❏	_____
15. Place towel or waterproof pad across patient's chest	❏	❏	_____
16. Instruct patient to take deep breath and hold it; pinch tube with fingers or clamp; quickly and smoothly remove tube while patient is holding breath	❏	❏	_____
17. Provide patient with tissues to cleanse nasal passage	❏	❏	_____
18. Place tubing in plastic bag or towel	❏	❏	_____
19. Cleanse nose with alcohol to remove residue from nasal guard placement	❏	❏	_____
20. Provide oral and nasal care; make patient comfortable	❏	❏	_____
21. Dispose of tube and equipment; measure drainage; note color and write down for documentation	❏	❏	_____

Postprocedure

	S	U	Comments
22. Assist patient to a position of comfort and place needed items within easy reach; be certain patient has a means to call for assistance and knows how to use it	❏	❏	_____
23. Raise the side rails and lower the bed to the lowest position	❏	❏	_____
24. Palpate abdomen periodically, noting any distention, pain, and rigidity; auscultate abdomen for bowel sounds	❏	❏	_____
25. Remove gloves and all protective barriers and/or remove and dispose of soiled supplies and equipment	❏	❏	_____
26. Wash hands after patient contact and after removing gloves	❏	❏	_____
27. Document and do patient teaching	❏	❏	_____
28. Report any unexpected outcomes	❏	❏	_____

PERFORMANCE CHECKLIST 19-26

Administering an Enema

	S	U	Comments

Prepare for procedure

1. Refer to medical record, care plan, or Kardex ❑ ❑ _____

2. Introduce self ❑ ❑ _____

3. Identify patient ❑ ❑ _____

4. Explain the procedure and the reason it is to be done ❑ ❑ _____

5. Assess need for and provide patient teaching during procedure ❑ ❑ _____

6. Assess patient ❑ ❑ _____

7. Wash hands and don clean gloves ❑ ❑ _____

8. Assemble equipment and complete necessary charges ❑ ❑ _____

9. Prepare patient for intervention

    a. Close door/pull privacy curtain ❑ ❑ _____

    b. Raise bed to comfortable working height; lower side rail on side nearest the nurse ❑ ❑ _____

    c. Position and drape patient as necessary ❑ ❑ _____

During the skill:

10. Promote patient involvement as possible ❑ ❑ _____

11. Assess patient's tolerance ❑ ❑ _____

12. Prepare solution ❑ ❑ _____

13. Arrange equipment at bedside; assist patient to the Sims' position ❑ ❑ _____

14. When giving an enema to a patient who is unable to contract the external sphincter, position the patient on the bedpan ❑ ❑ _____

	S	U	Comments
15. Place waterproof pad under patient	❏	❏	_____
16. Place bath blanket over patient and fan-fold linen to foot of bed; adjust patient's gown	❏	❏	_____
17. Clamp tubing 28 cm (7 in) from end; fill container with correctly warmed solution (usually 1000 ml at 105° F for adults) and any additives; allow solution to fill tubing to prevent air in colon	❏	❏	_____
18. For commercially prepared enema	❏	❏	_____
a. Remove cover from tip of enema; add additional lubricant and insert entire tip into anus; squeeze container until it is empty	❏	❏	_____
b. Lubricate tubing; spread patient's buttocks to expose anus; while rotating tube, gently insert it 7–10 cm (3–4 in); instruct patient to breathe out slowly through mouth	❏	❏	_____
c. Elevate container 30–45 cm (12–18 in) above level of anus	❏	❏	_____
d. Release clamp; allow more solution to flow slowly while holding clamp	❏	❏	_____
e. Lower container or clamp tubing if patient complains of cramping; encourage slow, deep breathing (when severe cramping, bleeding, or sudden abdominal pain occurs that is unrelieved by temporarily stopping or slowing flow of solution, stop enema and notify physician)	❏	❏	_____
f. Clamp and remove tube when all of the solution has been administered; encourage patient to retain solution at least 5 minutes	❏	❏	_____
19. When patient can no longer retain solution, assist to bedpan, bedside commode, or bathroom	❏	❏	_____
20. Instruct patient to call for nurse to inspect results before flushing stool; observe characteristics of feces/solution	❏	❏	_____
21. Provide for patient hygiene	❏	❏	_____

	S	U	Comments

Postprocedure

22. Assist patient to a position of comfort and place needed items within easy reach; be certain patient has a means to call for assistance and knows how to use it ❑ ❑ _____

23. Raise the side rails and lower the bed to the lowest position ❑ ❑ _____

24. Remove gloves and all protective barriers and/or remove and dispose of soiled supplies and equipment appropriately ❑ ❑ _____

25. Wash hands after patient contact and after removing gloves; provide for patient hygiene and assist patient to the bed or to the chair ❑ ❑ _____

26. Document and do patient teaching ❑ ❑ _____

27. Report any unexpected outcomes ❑ ❑ _____

PERFORMANCE CHECKLIST 19-27

DIGITAL EXAMINATION WITH REMOVAL OF FECAL IMPACTION

	S	U	Comments

Prepare for procedure

1. Refer to medical record, care plan, or Kardex   ❏   ❏   _____

2. Introduce self   ❏   ❏   _____

3. Identify patient   ❏   ❏   _____

4. Explain the procedure and the reason it is to be done   ❏   ❏   _____

5. Assess need for and provide patient teaching during procedure   ❏   ❏   _____

6. Assess patient   ❏   ❏   _____

7. Wash hands and don clean gloves   ❏   ❏   _____

8. Assemble equipment and complete necessary charges   ❏   ❏   _____

9. Prepare patient for intervention

     a. Close door/pull privacy curtain   ❏   ❏   _____

     b. Raise bed to comfortable working height; lower side rail on side nearest the nurse   ❏   ❏   _____

     c. Position and drape patient as necessary   ❏   ❏   _____

During the skill:

10. Promote patient involvement as possible   ❏   ❏   _____

11. Assess patient's tolerance   ❏   ❏   _____

12. Assist patient to assume the Sims' position and place waterproof pad under patient's buttocks   ❏   ❏   _____

13. Place the bedpan on the bed close to the patient's buttocks   ❏   ❏   _____

14. Don gloves; lubricate forefinger well with petroleum or water-soluble lubricant; use the index finger of your dominant hand   ❏   ❏   _____

	S	U	Comments
15. Insert finger gently; slowly but gently move finger into and around the fecal mass; as pieces of the mass are broken off, remove them to bedpan	❑	❑	_____
16. Instruct patient to take slow, deep breaths	❑	❑	_____
17. Continue procedure until impaction is removed	❑	❑	_____
18. Stop procedure for a few minutes if patient complains of severe discomfort; give patient opportunity to rest. Be alert for complications such as adverse vagal response	❑	❑	_____
19. After removal is complete, wash and dry perineal area	❑	❑	_____
20. Assist the patient to toilet or position on the bedpan if urge to defecate develops	❑	❑	_____

Postprocedure

	S	U	Comments
21. Assist patient to a position of comfort and place needed items within easy reach; be certain patient has a means to call for assistance and knows how to use it	❑	❑	_____
22. Raise the side rails and lower the bed to the lowest position	❑	❑	_____
23. Remove gloves and all protective barriers and/or remove and dispose of soiled supplies and equipment appropriately	❑	❑	_____
24. Wash hands after patient contact and after removing gloves	❑	❑	_____
25. Document and do patient teaching	❑	❑	_____
26. Report any unexpected outcomes	❑	❑	_____

PERFORMANCE CHECKLIST 19-28

Performing Colostomy, Ileostomy, and Urostomy Care

	S	U	Comments
Prepare for procedure			
1. Refer to medical record, care plan, or Kardex	❏	❏	_____
2. Introduce self	❏	❏	_____
3. Identify patient	❏	❏	_____
4. Explain the procedure and the reason it is to be done	❏	❏	_____
5. Assess need for and provide patient teaching during procedure	❏	❏	_____
6. Assess patient	❏	❏	_____
7. Wash hands and don clean gloves	❏	❏	_____
8. Assemble equipment and complete necessary charges	❏	❏	_____
9. Prepare patient for intervention			
a. Close door/pull privacy curtain	❏	❏	_____
b. Raise bed to comfortable working height; lower side rail on side nearest the nurse	❏	❏	_____
c. Position and drape patient as necessary	❏	❏	_____
During the skill:			
10. Promote patient involvement as possible	❏	❏	_____
11. Assess patient's tolerance	❏	❏	_____
12. Arrange supplies/equipment at bedside or in bathroom	❏	❏	_____
13. Position patient supine and make comfortable	❏	❏	_____
14. Unfasten and remove belt, if worn; carefully remove wafer seal from skin	❏	❏	_____
15. Place reusable pouch in bedpan or disposable pouch in plastic bag. Place bag away from patient to prevent unpleasant odors	❏	❏	_____

		S	**U**	**Comments**
16.	Cleanse skin with warm water; pat dry	❏	❏	_____
17.	Measure stoma using measuring device	❏	❏	_____
18.	Place toilet tissue or disposable wash cloth over stoma; use gauze for ileostomy; if using Skin Prep, apply to skin and allow to dry	❏	❏	_____
19.	Apply protective skin barrier about $\frac{1}{16}$ inch from stoma; assess stoma to determine color and viability	❏	❏	_____
20.	Apply protective wafer with flange, cutting an opening in the center of wafer to $\frac{1}{16}$ inch larger than stoma	❏	❏	_____
21.	Gently attach pouch to flange by compressing the two together (a new device is available called Autolok which snaps into place with a smooth lock, thus eliminating the need to compress the flange to the pouch)	❏	❏	_____
22.	Remove tissue or gauze from stoma and backing from protectant; center opening over stoma and press against skin for 1–2 minutes	❏	❏	_____
23.	Fold bottom edges of pouch over one time to fit clamp	❏	❏	_____
24.	Secure clamp	❏	❏	_____
25.	If belt is used, attach properly	❏	❏	_____
26.	Assist patient to comfortable position in bed or chair; remove equipment from bedside	❏	❏	_____
27.	Empty, wash, and dry reusable pouch	❏	❏	_____

Urostomy care

		S	**U**	**Comments**
28.	Follow steps 1 to 13 of ostomy care procedure	❏	❏	_____
29.	Empty urine into graduated pitcher; write down amount and characteristics of urine for later documentation (mucus will be present in urine from shedding of mucus by mucous membrane of intestine as urine passes over the intestinal conduit)	❏	❏	_____

	S	U	Comments
30. Carefully remove water seal from skin and place pouch in plastic bag	❏	❏	_____
31. Cleanse skin with warm water and pat dry	❏	❏	_____
32. Measure stoma using measuring device	❏	❏	_____
33. Place gauze over stoma	❏	❏	_____
34. If using Skin Prep, apply to skin and allow to dry; apply protective stoma paste about $\frac{1}{16}$ inch from the stoma	❏	❏	_____
35. Apply protective wafer with flange, cutting an opening in the center of wafer $\frac{1}{16}$ inch larger than stoma; assess stoma to determine color and viability	❏	❏	_____

Postprocedure

	S	U	Comments
36. Assist patient to a position of comfort and place needed items within easy reach; be certain patient has a means to call for assistance and knows how to use it	❏	❏	_____
37. Raise the side rails and lower the bed to the lowest position	❏	❏	_____
38. Remove gloves and all protective barriers and/or remove and dispose of soiled supplies and equipment appropriately	❏	❏	_____
39. Wash hands after patient contact and after removing gloves	❏	❏	_____
40. Document and do patient teaching	❏	❏	_____
41. Report any unexpected outcomes	❏	❏	_____

PERFORMANCE CHECKLIST 19-29

PERFORMING A COLOSTOMY IRRIGATION

		S	**U**	**Comments**
Prepare for procedure				
1.	Refer to medical record, care plan, or Kardex	❏	❏	_____
2.	Introduce self	❏	❏	_____
3.	Identify patient	❏	❏	_____
4.	Explain the procedure and the reason it is to be done	❏	❏	_____
5.	Assess need for and provide patient teaching during procedure	❏	❏	_____
6.	Assess patient	❏	❏	_____
7.	Wash hands and don clean gloves	❏	❏	_____
8.	Assemble equipment and complete necessary charges	❏	❏	_____
9.	Prepare patient for intervention			
a.	Close door/pull privacy curtain	❏	❏	_____
b.	Raise bed to comfortable working height; lower side rail on side nearest the nurse	❏	❏	_____
c.	Position and drape patient as necessary	❏	❏	_____
During the skill:				
10.	Promote patient involvement as possible	❏	❏	_____
11.	Assess patient's tolerance	❏	❏	_____
12.	Position patient			
a.	Bathroom: instruct patient to sit on toilet or on a chair in front of the toilet	❏	❏	_____
b.	Bed: have patient lie comfortably with head of bed slightly elevated	❏	❏	_____

	S	U	Comments

NOTE: As many of the following steps as possible should be performed by the patient with the nurse teaching and assisting as needed; independence will come; be alert to patient readiness

13. Remove pouch, cleanse skin, and place irrigation sleeve over stoma; attach belt if using; place end of sleeve in toilet ❏ ❏ _____

14. Close clamp on irrigating tubing; fill irrigating container with 1000 ml tepid water (or as otherwise ordered); container may be hung on a hook at patient's shoulder level ❏ ❏ _____

15. Allow a small amount of water to flow through tubing ❏ ❏ _____

16. Attach cone to tubing; lubricate cone; gently insert cone into stoma through top of sleeve ❏ ❏ _____

17. While holding cone in place, allow solution to flow slowly into colon (500–1000 ml over 15 minutes) ❏ ❏ _____

18. After all solution is instilled, remove cone and close top of sleeve ❏ ❏ _____

19. Instruct patient to sit about 15–20 minutes while returns flow into toilet ❏ ❏ _____

20. Drain sleeve; remove and rinse it ❏ ❏ _____

21. Observe patient and results of irrigation; flush toilet ❏ ❏ _____

22. Perform colostomy care ❏ ❏ _____

Postprocedure

23. Assist patient to a position of comfort and place needed items within easy reach; be certain patient has a means to call for assistance and knows how to use it ❏ ❏ _____

24. Raise the side rails and lower the bed to the lowest position ❏ ❏ _____

		S	U	Comments
25.	Remove gloves and all protective barriers and/or remove and dispose of soiled supplies and equipment appropriately	❏	❏	_____
26.	Wash hands after patient contact and after removing gloves	❏	❏	_____
27.	Document and do patient teaching	❏	❏	_____
28.	Report any unexpected outcomes	❏	❏	_____

PERFORMANCE CHECKLIST 19-30

PERFORMING A NASAL IRRIGATION

	S	U	Comments
1. Refer to medical record, care plan or Kardex for special interventions	❏	❏	_____
2. Obtain equipment and assemble	❏	❏	_____
3. Wash hands	❏	❏	_____
4. Introduce self	❏	❏	_____
5. Identify patient	❏	❏	_____
6. Explain procedure	❏	❏	_____
7. Assess patient for comfort level and any nasal secretions, don gloves as necessary; if gloves are worn, remove, dispose of appropriately, and wash hands	❏	❏	_____
8. Prepare patient			
a. Provide privacy	❏	❏	_____
b. Position patient sitting upright comfortably near equipment leaning over the basin or sink	❏	❏	_____
9. Prepare equipment			
a. Mix solution as needed	❏	❏	_____
b. Warm solution	❏	❏	_____
c. Fill irrigating device	❏	❏	_____
d. Place basin as collecting receptacle	❏	❏	_____
10. Don gloves	❏	❏	_____
11. Instruct patient to keep mouth open and breathe rhythmically during procedure	❏	❏	_____
12. Teach patient neither to speak nor swallow during procedure	❏	❏	_____

	S	U	Comments
13. Remove irrigating device tip from nose if patient reports the need to cough or sneeze	❏	❏	_____
14. Perform procedure			
a. Oral irrigating device			
(1) Insert tip about ½ to 1 inch into patient's nostril	❏	❏	_____
(2) Begin with a low pressure setting	❏	❏	_____
(3) Irrigate both nostrils	❏	❏	_____
b. Bulb syringe			
(1) Insert tip ½ inch into patient's nostril	❏	❏	_____
(2) Squeeze bulb until a gentle stream of warm solution washes through the nose	❏	❏	_____
(3) Avoid forceful squeezing	❏	❏	_____
(4) Irrigate both nostrils until returns are clear	❏	❏	_____
15. Assess returns and report any abnormalities			
a. Color	❏	❏	_____
b. Viscosity	❏	❏	_____
c. Volume	❏	❏	_____
d. Blood	❏	❏	_____
e. Necrotic material	❏	❏	_____

Postprocedure

	S	U	Comments
16. Request patient to wait a few minutes before blowing nose	❏	❏	_____
17. Instruct patient to gently blow both nostrils at the same time	❏	❏	_____
18. Clean and store equipment	❏	❏	_____

		S	**U**	**Comments**
19.	Remove gloves, dispose of appropriately and wash hands	❏	❏	_____
20.	Assist patient to cleanse and dry self	❏	❏	_____
21.	Assist to bed or chair; make certain of patient's comfort and place needed items within reach	❏	❏	_____
22.	If in bed raise side rail and lower bed to lowest position	❏	❏	_____
23.	Wash hands	❏	❏	_____
24.	Document	❏	❏	_____
25.	Observe and assess patient for any adverse reactions	❏	❏	_____
26.	Do patient teaching	❏	❏	_____

PERFORMANCE CHECKLIST 20-1

Administering Nasogastric Tube Feedings

	S	U	Comments
1. Refer to medical record, care plan, or Kardex for special interventions	❏	❏	_____
2. Obtain equipment and assemble	❏	❏	_____
3. Wash hands	❏	❏	_____
4. Don gloves	❏	❏	_____
5. Introduce self	❏	❏	_____
6. Identify patient	❏	❏	_____
7. Explain procedure	❏	❏	_____
8. Assess patient, auscultate for active bowel sounds to assess abdomen for distention or tenderness	❏	❏	_____
9. Prepare patient; close door to room, pull privacy curtain	❏	❏	_____
10. Raise bed to a comfortable working height	❏	❏	_____
11. Elevate level of bed to Fowler's, at least 30 degrees, or reverse Trendelenburg if spinal injury present	❏	❏	_____
12. Check for placement of feeding tube:			
a. By x-ray	❏	❏	_____
b. By aspiration of gastric contents with a cone-tipped syringe	❏	❏	_____
c. By testing the pH to determine acid pH; place drop of GI contents on pH test paper (gastric content should have a pH of 0–4, tracheobronchial and pleural secretions should have a pH > 6 and intestinal contents usually have a pH of 7 or greater)	❏	❏	_____
d. Inspect oral cavity for tube kinking or curling in back of throat	❏	❏	_____

		S	U	Comments

e. If unable to aspirate, consider tube is occluded or kinked, and attempt to flush with 30 ml of warm water ❏ ❏ _____

13. Readminister residual volume to patient slowly ❏ ❏ _____

    a. If residual amounts are greater than last infusion or 150 ml, hold feeding for one hour and reassess residual ❏ ❏ _____

14. Prepare formula for administration ❏ ❏ _____

15. Bolus or intermittent feedings:

    a. Administer tube feeding with 60 ml bulb or plunger syringe ❏ ❏ _____

    b. Remove cap or plug from end of feeding tube and pinch closed ❏ ❏ _____

    c. Attach syringe by removing bulb or plunger and inserting tip into end of tube. Elevate to no more than 18 inches above insertion site ❏ ❏ _____

    d. Fill syringe with formula, release tube, and allow syringe to empty gradually, refilling until prescribed ordered amount has been administered ❏ ❏ _____

    e. Flush tube with 30–60 ml tap water ❏ ❏ _____

    f. Recap/plug tube ❏ ❏ _____

16. Continuous drip method:

    a. Administer tube feeding with gavage bag ❏ ❏ _____

    b. Prepare administration set: clamp tubing, prepare gavage bag with prescribed type and amount of formula, unclamp and prime tubing to remove air, then reclamp tubing ❏ ❏ _____

    c. Label bag with tube feeding type, strength, and amount. Include date, time, and initials ❏ ❏ _____

		S	**U**	**Comments**

d. Pinch end of feeding tube. Remove plug/cap and securely attach gavage tubing to end of feeding tube ❏ ❏ _____

e. Set rate by adjusting roller clamp on tubing ❏ ❏ _____

f. Flush tube with 30–60 ml tap water ❏ ❏ _____

g. Recap/plug tube ❏ ❏ _____

17. Feeding via infusion pump:

a. Administer tube feeding as a continuous drip via infusion pump ❏ ❏ _____

b. Prepare administration set. Clamp tubing, spike bag, unclamp and prime tubing. Reclamp tubing ❏ ❏ _____

c. Label bag with tube feeding type, strength, and amount. Include date, time, and initials ❏ ❏ _____

d. Hang tube feeding set on IV pole with infusion pump. Connect tubing to pump and set rate ❏ ❏ _____

e. Pinch end of feeding tube. Remove plug/cap. Connect infusion tubing to patient feeding tube ❏ ❏ _____

f. Open roller clamp on infusion tubing ❏ ❏ _____

g. Check residual volumes every 4 hours ❏ ❏ _____

18. Fill a 60 ml syringe with ordered volume of water (30–50 ml). Inject into feeding tube to flush after bolus or as ordered with continuous drip ❏ ❏ _____

19. Flush tube with water every 4–8 hours, clamp it when no feedings are infusing ❏ ❏ _____

20. Rinse syringe or bag and tubing with warm water. Remove and discard gloves and wash hands ❏ ❏ _____

21. Assist patient to a position of comfort and place needed items within reach ❏ ❏ _____

		S	U	Comments
22.	Raise side rails and lower bed to lowest position	❏	❏	_____
23.	Remove gloves, dispose of used supplies and wash hands	❏	❏	_____
24.	Document	❏	❏	_____
25.	Monitor weight and laboratory values daily	❏	❏	_____
26.	Observe and assess patient for any adverse reaction	❏	❏	_____

PERFORMANCE CHECKLIST 20-2

Administering Enteral Feedings Via Gastrostomy or Jejunostomy Tube

	S	U	Comments

Observe all guidelines for nasal gastric tube feedings and follow steps 1 to 11 of Skill 20-1 and then continue with the steps below.

1. Verify tube placement—see Skill 20-1, step 12

   a. Gastrostomy tube: aspirate gastric secretions, check pH; return aspirated contents to stomach unless volume exceeds 150 ml ❏ ❏ _____

   b. Jejunostomy tube: aspirate intestinal secretions, check pH ❏ ❏ _____

2. Flush with 30 ml water ❏ ❏ _____

3. Initiate feedings:

   a. Syringe feedings:

      (1) Pinch proximal end of gastrostomy tube ❏ ❏ _____

      (2) Remove plunger and attach barrel of syringe to end of tube, then fill syringe with formula ❏ ❏ _____

      (3) Allow syringe to empty gradually. Refill until prescribed amount has been delivered to patient ❏ ❏ _____

      (4) Flush with ordered volume of water (30–50 ml) ❏ ❏ _____

   b. Continuous drip method:

      (1) Fill feeding container with enough formula for 4 hrs of feeding ❏ ❏ _____

      (2) Hang container on IV pole, and clear tubing of air ❏ ❏ _____

      (3) Thread tubing on pump according to manufacturer's directions ❏ ❏ _____

		S	U	Comments
(4)	Connect tubing to end of feeding tube	❏	❏	_____
(5)	Begin infusion at prescribed rate	❏	❏	_____
4.	Assess skin around tube exit site	❏	❏	_____
5.	Dispose of supplies and wash hands	❏	❏	_____
6.	Monitor finger-stick blood glucose every 6 hrs until maximum administration rate is reached and maintained for 24 hrs	❏	❏	_____
7.	Monitor intake and output	❏	❏	_____
8.	Weigh patient daily	❏	❏	_____
9.	Observe laboratory values	❏	❏	_____
10.	Inspect enteral site for signs of pressure	❏	❏	_____
11.	Document	❏	❏	_____

PERFORMANCE CHECKLIST 21-1

Measuring Intake and Output (I&O)

		S	U	Comments
1.	Read physician's order	❑	❑	_____
2.	Identify patient	❑	❑	_____
3.	Explain procedure	❑	❑	_____
4.	Instruct patient to inform staff of all oral intake	❑	❑	_____
5.	Provide a marked I&O container	❑	❑	_____
6.	Instruct patient not to empty any output collection receptacles and to notify the nurse after elimination	❑	❑	_____
7.	Post signs on patient's door, bathroom door, and near patient's bed	❑	❑	_____
8.	Measure and record all fluids taken orally or per feeding tube, and all fluids administered parenterally	❑	❑	_____
9.	Wash hands and don gloves	❑	❑	_____
10.	Measure and record output in urinary drainage system, diarrhea stools, nasogastric suction, emesis, and output in surgical wound receptacles such as Davol, Jackson-Pratt, and Hemovac	❑	❑	_____
11.	Remove gloves and wash hands	❑	❑	_____
12.	Compute and document I&O on patient's record	❑	❑	_____
13.	Be vigilant to maintain accurate I&O when ordered	❑	❑	_____

Student Name _____ Date _____ Instructor's Name _____

PERFORMANCE CHECKLIST 22-1

ADMINISTERING TABLETS, PILLS, AND CAPSULES

		S	U	Comments
1.	Follow the six rights	❑	❑	_____
2.	Perform the three label checks	❑	❑	_____
3.	Follow standard precautions	❑	❑	_____
4.	Wash hands	❑	❑	_____
5.	Check for allergies	❑	❑	_____
6.	If using unit dose package, place unopened package in medicine cup	❑	❑	_____
7.	If using a multidose bottle, pour tablet into cap of bottle appropriately	❑	❑	_____
8.	Pour tablet from cap into medicine cup	❑	❑	_____
9.	If using medicine tray (for several patients), set it up from left to right, front to back	❑	❑	_____
10.	If pouring from multidose bottle and patient is to receive several tablets, use separate cup for medications such as digitalis. If the patient's pulse is less than 60/min, withhold the medication and report this to the RN. Place digitalis in a separate cup marked with a red heart to allow for easy identification	❑	❑	_____
11.	Do not use pills, tablets, or capsules that come from multidose bottles if they have been handled or dropped on the floor	❑	❑	_____
12.	Take medication to the room	❑	❑	_____
13.	Follow procedure for room, bed, and patient identification	❑	❑	_____
14.	Check again for allergies	❑	❑	_____

	S	U	Comments
15. Explain procedure to patient	❏	❏	_____
16. Document	❏	❏	_____
17. Return to assess patient	❏	❏	_____
18. Document assessment	❏	❏	_____

Student Name _____ Date _____ Instructor's Name _____

PERFORMANCE CHECKLIST 22-2

Administering Liquid Medications

	S	U	Comments
1. Follow the six rights	❑	❑	_____
2. Perform the three label checks	❑	❑	_____
3. Follow standard precautions	❑	❑	_____
4. Wash hands	❑	❑	_____
5. Check for allergies	❑	❑	_____
6. Remove liquid preparation from patient's drug box/bin (or from medication cabinet or refrigerator)	❑	❑	_____
7. Check dosage/ml and total volume of medication in container	❑	❑	_____
8. Calculate dosage; if the dosage ordered is different from the dosage/ml stated on the label, calculate correct dose; if ordered medication is labeled in a different measurement system, convert by using appropriate equivalent. Work problem on paper correctly	❑	❑	_____
9. Check calculations with another nurse	❑	❑	_____
10. Obtain graduated medicine cup or appropriate syringe	❑	❑	_____
11. Face label of bottle toward palm of hand to avoid soiling label; if label becomes soiled, return the bottle to the pharmacy; do not give medication if label is unreadable	❑	❑	_____
12. Place medicine cup on flat surface, or hold at eye level while pouring	❑	❑	_____
13. Place cap of bottle with inner rim up	❑	❑	_____
14. Read dosage amount at lower level of meniscus	❑	❑	_____
15. Transport medication to patient's room	❑	❑	_____

		S	U	Comments
16.	Follow procedure for room, bed, and patient identification	❏	❏	_____
17.	Check for allergies again	❏	❏	_____
18.	Explain procedure to patient	❏	❏	_____
19.	Document administration in the correct manner	❏	❏	_____
20.	Return to assess patient	❏	❏	_____
21.	Document assessment	❏	❏	_____

PERFORMANCE CHECKLIST 22-3

Administering Tubal Medications

		S	U	Comments
1.	Follow the six rights	❏	❏	_____
2.	Perform the three label checks	❏	❏	_____
3.	Follow standard precautions	❏	❏	_____
4.	Wash hands	❏	❏	_____
5.	Check for allergies	❏	❏	_____
6.	Prepare medication using the same procedure as for liquid medications	❏	❏	_____
7.	If tablet, crush pill, dissolve in 15–20 ml warm water. For capsules, open and dissolve powder in 15–30 ml warm water. For gelatin capsules, aspirate with syringe or capsule may be dissolved in warm water and remove gelatin outer layer	❏	❏	_____
8.	Gather equipment	❏	❏	_____
9.	Take equipment and medication to patient's room	❏	❏	_____
10.	Follow procedure of room, bed, and patient identification	❏	❏	_____
11.	Recheck for allergies	❏	❏	_____
12.	Explain procedure; answer questions patient may have about the procedure	❏	❏	_____
13.	Place patient in high Fowler's position	❏	❏	_____
14.	Put towel over patient's chest	❏	❏	_____
15.	Don disposable, unsterile gloves	❏	❏	_____
16.	Check and recheck placement and patency of tube with the appropriate procedure	❏	❏	_____
17.	Clamp tube appropriately	❏	❏	_____

		S	U	Comments
18.	Attach syringe to end of tube correctly	❏	❏	_____
19.	Pour medication into syringe	❏	❏	_____
20.	Unclamp tubing to allow medication to slowly flow by gravity	❏	❏	_____
21.	Follow medication with 30–50 ml of water	❏	❏	_____
22.	Clamp tubing; secure tube after medication is given	❏	❏	_____
23.	If NG tube is attached to suction, do not reconnect suction for 30 minutes	❏	❏	_____
24.	Remove towel from patient	❏	❏	_____
25.	Remove gloves and dispose of properly	❏	❏	_____
26.	Leave patient in comfortable position	❏	❏	_____
27.	Gather equipment; clean up patient and area appropriately	❏	❏	_____
28.	Wash hands	❏	❏	_____
29.	Document	❏	❏	_____
30.	Return to assess patient	❏	❏	_____
31.	Document assessment	❏	❏	_____

PERFORMANCE CHECKLIST 22-4

Administering Rectal Suppositories

		S	U	Comments
1.	Follow the six rights	❏	❏	_____
2.	Perform the three label checks	❏	❏	_____
3.	Follow standard precautions	❏	❏	_____
4.	Wash hands	❏	❏	_____
5.	Check for allergies	❏	❏	_____
6.	Obtain water-soluble lubricant	❏	❏	_____
7.	Obtain suppository	❏	❏	_____
8.	Place unopened suppository into medicine cup or souffle cup	❏	❏	_____
9.	Take disposable, unsterile gloves or finger cot to room	❏	❏	_____
10.	Follow procedure of room, bed, and patient identification	❏	❏	_____
11.	Explain procedure to patient	❏	❏	_____
12.	Gain patient's cooperation	❏	❏	_____
13.	Provide privacy	❏	❏	_____
14.	Position patient appropriately (Sims' position)	❏	❏	_____
15.	Unwrap suppository	❏	❏	_____
16.	Maintain privacy; expose buttocks	❏	❏	_____
17.	Don gloves	❏	❏	_____
18.	Apply lubricant	❏	❏	_____
19.	Ask patient to take deep breath; insert beyond internal anal sphincter	❏	❏	_____

		S	U	Comments
20.	Ask patient to retain suppository as long as possible; hold the buttocks together to help patient to retain suppository	❏	❏	_____
21.	Discard gloves correctly	❏	❏	_____
22.	Help patient assume comfortable position	❏	❏	_____
23.	Wash hands	❏	❏	_____
24.	Document	❏	❏	_____
25.	Return to assess patient	❏	❏	_____
26.	Document assessment	❏	❏	_____

PERFORMANCE CHECKLIST 22-5

Applying Topical Agents

		S	U	Comments
1.	Follow the six rights	❏	❏	_____
2.	Perform the three label checks	❏	❏	_____
3.	Follow standard precautions	❏	❏	_____
4.	Wash hands	❏	❏	_____
5.	Check for allergies	❏	❏	_____
6.	Transport medication to room	❏	❏	_____
7.	Identify room, bed, and patient	❏	❏	_____
8.	Recheck for allergies	❏	❏	_____
9.	Introduce self; explain procedure to patient	❏	❏	_____
10.	Provide privacy; place patient in comfortable position that allows exposure to selected site	❏	❏	_____
11.	Cleanse site with appropriate materials	❏	❏	_____
12.	Don gloves	❏	❏	_____
13.	Read prescription instructions carefully	❏	❏	_____
14.	Prepare medicinal agent (ointments, creams, and lotions may have to be squeezed or removed with a tongue blade, depending on preparation)	❏	❏	_____
15.	Apply paper applicator, disk, lotion, ointment, or cream	❏	❏	_____
16.	Remove gloves	❏	❏	_____
17.	Leave patient properly draped or clothed in comfortable position	❏	❏	_____

	S	U	Comments
18. Answer patient's questions, and teach patient to perform self-applications if appropriate	❑	❑	_____
19. Clean work area	❑	❑	_____
20. Wash hands	❑	❑	_____
21. Document administration	❑	❑	_____
22. Return to assess patient	❑	❑	_____
23. Document assessment	❑	❑	_____

PERFORMANCE CHECKLIST 22-6

ADMINISTERING EYEDROPS AND EYE OINTMENTS

	S	U	Comments
1. Follow the six rights	❏	❏	_____
2. Perform the three label checks	❏	❏	_____
3. Follow standard precautions	❏	❏	_____
4. Wash hands	❏	❏	_____
5. Check for allergies	❏	❏	_____
6. Transport medications to room	❏	❏	_____
7. Identify medications as ophthalmic	❏	❏	_____
8. Identify room, bed, and patient	❏	❏	_____
9. Recheck for allergies	❏	❏	_____
10. Introduce self; explain procedure	❏	❏	_____
11. Provide privacy, position back of patient's head on pillow; direct patient's face upward toward ceiling. Review which eye or eyes to receive the medication; OS = left eye, OD = right eye, OU = each eye	❏	❏	_____
12. Recheck for allergies	❏	❏	_____
13. Don gloves	❏	❏	_____
14. Remove exudate; clean eye as needed using sterile solution of saline; use cotton balls to wipe away exudate; use one cotton ball per stroke, wiping from inner canthus outward	❏	❏	_____
15. To apply drops, expose lower conjunctival sac by having patient look upward while gentle traction is applied to lower eyelid	❏	❏	_____
16. Put prescribed number of drops into conjunctival sac, not onto eyeball	❏	❏	_____

		S	U	Comments
17.	Using a cotton ball or tissue, apply gentle pressure above bone at inner corner of eyelid for 1–2 minutes	❑	❑	_____
18.	Apply sterile dressing if ordered	❑	❑	_____
19.	To apply ointment, expose lower conjunctival sac by having patient look upward while gentle traction is applied to lower eyelid	❑	❑	_____
20.	Squeeze ointment into lower conjunctival sac	❑	❑	_____
21.	Ask patient to close eye and to move it around in circular motion to spread medication	❑	❑	_____
22.	Apply sterile dressing if ordered	❑	❑	_____
23.	After applying drops or ointment to an eye, leave patient in comfortable position; clean up the work area	❑	❑	_____
24.	Remove gloves and wash hands	❑	❑	_____
25.	Answer patient's questions and if appropriate, teach patient to perform self-care	❑	❑	_____
26.	Record administration of medications in Medex or computer with initials, date, and time	❑	❑	_____
27.	Return to assess patient's response to medication	❑	❑	_____
28.	Document assessment in nurse's notes	❑	❑	_____

PERFORMANCE CHECKLIST 22-7

ADMINISTERING EARDROPS

		S	U	Comments
1.	Follow the six rights	❏	❏	_____
2.	Perform the three label checks	❏	❏	_____
3.	Follow standard precautions	❏	❏	_____
4.	Wash hands	❏	❏	_____
5.	Check for allergies	❏	❏	_____
6.	Transport medication to room	❏	❏	_____
7.	Identify medications as otic	❏	❏	_____
8.	Identify room, bed, and patient	❏	❏	_____
9.	Recheck for allergies	❏	❏	_____
10.	Introduce self; explain procedure	❏	❏	_____
11.	Provide privacy; position patient with affected ear upward	❏	❏	_____
12.	Don gloves	❏	❏	_____
13.	Remove external exudate from ear; an order must be obtained before irrigating the ear	❏	❏	_____
14.	Draw medication into dropper	❏	❏	_____
15.	For adults and for children over 3 years old, turn head with affected side up; pull earlobe upward and back to straighten external auditory canal; give drops without touching ear with dropper	❏	❏	_____
16.	For children under 3 years old, turn head with affected side up; pull earlobe downward and back; instill drops without touching ear with dropper	❏	❏	_____

	S	U	Comments
17. Tell patient to remain in same position for a few minutes to allow medication to drain into ear by gravity	❏	❏	_____
18. A cotton ball may be placed loosely into ear as needed	❏	❏	_____
19. Remove gloves	❏	❏	_____
20. Leave patient in comfortable position; clean work area	❏	❏	_____
21. Answer patient's questions and if appropriate, teach patient self-care	❏	❏	_____
22. Wash hands	❏	❏	_____
23. Record administration in Medex or computer with initials, date, and time	❏	❏	_____
24. Return to assess patient's response to medication	❏	❏	_____
25. Document assessment in nurse's notes	❏	❏	_____

PERFORMANCE CHECKLIST 22-8

ADMINISTERING NOSEDROPS

		S	U	Comments
1.	Follow the six rights	❑	❑	_____
2.	Perform the three label checks	❑	❑	_____
3.	Follow standard precautions	❑	❑	_____
4.	Wash hands	❑	❑	_____
5.	Check for allergies	❑	❑	_____
6.	Transport medication to room	❑	❑	_____
7.	Identify room, bed, and patient	❑	❑	_____
8.	Recheck for allergies	❑	❑	_____
9.	Introduce self; explain procedure	❑	❑	_____
10.	Provide privacy	❑	❑	_____
11.	Don gloves	❑	❑	_____
12.	Ask adult or older child to clear nose of accumulations by blowing gently into tissue	❑	❑	_____
13.	Have patient lie down, hanging head backward over edge of bed or with pillow under shoulders to hyperextend the neck if patient can tolerate it	❑	❑	_____
14.	After drawing medication into dropper, instill medication while holding dropper above nostril being treated	❑	❑	_____
15.	If ordered, repeat procedure to instill drops in other nostril	❑	❑	_____
16.	Tell patient to hold position for a few minutes to allow medication to remain in place	❑	❑	_____
17.	Administer nosedrops to a younger child after positioning him on bed with head backward and downward, or to an infant while holding his head backward and downward	❑	❑	_____

	S	U	Comments
18. Administer drops in same way as to an adult	❏	❏	_____
19. Remove gloves	❏	❏	_____
20. Tell patient to refrain from blowing nose immediately after instillation	❏	❏	_____
21. Offer tissues for later use	❏	❏	_____
22. Leave patient in comfortable position; clean work area	❏	❏	_____
23. Answer patient's questions and if appropriate, teach patient self-care	❏	❏	_____
24. Wash hands	❏	❏	_____
25. Record administration in Medex or computer with initials, date, and time	❏	❏	_____
26. Return to assess patient's response to medication	❏	❏	_____
27. Document assessment in nurse's notes	❏	❏	_____

PERFORMANCE CHECKLIST 22-9

ADMINISTERING NASAL SPRAYS

		S	U	Comments
1.	Follow the six rights	❏	❏	_____
2.	Perform the three label checks	❏	❏	_____
3.	Follow standard precautions	❏	❏	_____
4.	Wash hands	❏	❏	_____
5.	Check for allergies	❏	❏	_____
6.	Transport medication to patient	❏	❏	_____
7.	Identify room, bed, and patient	❏	❏	_____
8.	Recheck for allergies	❏	❏	_____
9.	Introduce self; explain procedure	❏	❏	_____
10.	Provide privacy; position patient upright	❏	❏	_____
11.	Don gloves	❏	❏	_____
12.	Determine which nostril (or both) is to receive the medications	❏	❏	_____
13.	Have patient gently blow nose to clear nasal passages of accumulations	❏	❏	_____
14.	Compress one nostril	❏	❏	_____
15.	Shake bottle while holding it upright	❏	❏	_____
16.	Insert tip of spray bottle into patient's patent nostril	❏	❏	_____
17.	Instruct patient to inhale; while he inhales, squeeze bottle	❏	❏	_____
18.	If ordered, repeat procedure for other nostril	❏	❏	_____
19.	Tell patient to refrain from blowing nose for a few minutes; offer tissues for later use	❏	❏	_____

	S	U	Comments
20. Answer patient's questions and if appropriate, teach self-administration	❑	❑	_____
21. Remove gloves and wash hands	❑	❑	_____
22. Record administration in Medex or computer with initials, date, and time	❑	❑	_____
23. Return to assess patient's response to medication	❑	❑	_____
24. Document assessment in nurse's notes	❑	❑	_____

PERFORMANCE CHECKLIST 22-10

ADMINISTERING INHALANTS

		S	U	Comments
1.	Follow the six rights	❏	❏	_____
2.	Perform the three label checks	❏	❏	_____
3.	Follow standard precautions	❏	❏	_____
4.	Wash hands	❏	❏	_____
5.	Check for allergies	❏	❏	_____
6.	Transport medication to patient	❏	❏	_____
7.	Identify room, bed, and patient	❏	❏	_____
8.	Recheck for allergies	❏	❏	_____
9.	Introduce self; explain procedure	❏	❏	_____
10.	Provide privacy	❏	❏	_____
11.	Allow patient opportunity to manipulate inhaler, canister, and spacer device (aerochamber); explain and demonstrate how canister fits into inhaler	❏	❏	_____
12.	Explain what metered dose is and warn patient about overuse of inhaler, including drug side effects	❏	❏	_____
13.	Remove mouthpiece cover from inhaler; shake inhaler well	❏	❏	_____
14.	*Without aerochamber (spacer):* Open lips and place inhaler 1–2 cm (½ to 1 inch) from mouth with opening toward back of throat. Lips should not touch inhaler	❏	❏	_____
15.	*With aerochamber (spacer):* Exhale fully, then grasp mouthpiece with teeth and lips while holding inhaler with thumb at the mouthpiece and fingers at the top	❏	❏	_____

		S	U	Comments
16.	Press down on inhaler to release medication while inhaling slowly and deeply through mouth	❏	❏	_____
17.	Breathe in slowly for 2–3 seconds; hold breath for approximately 10 seconds	❏	❏	_____
18.	Exhale through pursed lips	❏	❏	_____
19.	Instruct patient to wait 1 minute between puffs; more than one puff is usually prescribed	❏	❏	_____
20.	If more than one type of inhaled medications are prescribed, wait 5–10 minutes between inhalations or as ordered by physician	❏	❏	_____
21.	Explain that patient may feel gagging sensation in throat caused by droplets of medication on pharynx or tongue	❏	❏	_____
22.	Instruct patient in removing medication canister and cleaning inhaler in warm water	❏	❏	_____
23.	Teach patient to measure the amount of medication remaining in the canister by immersing it in a large bowl or pan of water	❏	❏	_____
24.	Record administration in Medex or computer with initials, date, and time	❏	❏	_____
25.	Return to assess patient's response to medication	❏	❏	_____
26.	Document assessment in nurse's notes	❏	❏	_____

PERFORMANCE CHECKLIST 22-11

Administering Sublingual Medication

		S	U	Comments
1.	Follow the six rights	❏	❏	_____
2.	Perform the three label checks	❏	❏	_____
3.	Follow standard precautions	❏	❏	_____
4.	Wash hands	❏	❏	_____
5.	Check for allergies	❏	❏	_____
6.	Identify room, bed, and patient	❏	❏	_____
7.	Recheck for allergies	❏	❏	_____
8.	Wear gloves to place tablet under patient's tongue	❏	❏	_____
9.	Do not follow with water	❏	❏	_____
10.	Instruct patient not to swallow tablet	❏	❏	_____
11.	Explain to patient how to place medication under tongue; instruct patient to let it dissolve	❏	❏	_____
12.	Remove gloves and wash hands	❏	❏	_____
13.	Document sublingual administration in Medex or computer with time, date, and initials	❏	❏	_____
14.	Return to assess patient's response to medication	❏	❏	_____
15.	Document assessment in nurse's notes	❏	❏	_____

PERFORMANCE CHECKLIST 22-12

ADMINISTERING BUCCAL MEDICATION

		S	U	Comments
1.	Follow the six rights	❏	❏	_____
2.	Perform the three label checks	❏	❏	_____
3.	Follow standard precautions	❏	❏	_____
4.	Wash hands	❏	❏	_____
5.	Check for allergies	❏	❏	_____
6.	Identify room, bed, and patient	❏	❏	_____
7.	Recheck for allergies	❏	❏	_____
8.	Wear gloves to place tablet between patient's cheek and gum	❏	❏	_____
9.	Do not follow with water	❏	❏	_____
10.	Instruct patient not to swallow tablet; let it dissolve	❏	❏	_____
11.	Explain to patient how to place medication between cheek and gum	❏	❏	_____
12.	Remove gloves and wash hands	❏	❏	_____
13.	Document buccal administration in Medex or computer with time, date, and initials	❏	❏	_____
14.	Return to assess patient's response to medication	❏	❏	_____
15.	Document assessment in nurse's notes	❏	❏	_____

PERFORMANCE CHECKLIST 22-13A

PREPARING PARENTERAL MEDICATIONS:
WITHDRAWING MEDICATION FROM A VIAL

		S	U	Comments
1.	Follow the six rights	❑	❑	_____
2.	Perform the three label checks	❑	❑	_____
3.	Follow standard precautions	❑	❑	_____
4.	Check for allergies	❑	❑	_____
5.	Wash hands before handling equipment; prepare medication in clean area; reduce distractions	❑	❑	_____
6.	Keep sterile parts of syringe and needle sterile; use aseptic technique throughout preparation	❑	❑	_____
7.	Compare drug and dosage ordered with drug and dosage on hand; check expiration date, dosage per milliliter, total volume of solution in vial; look for contaminants or defects in vial	❑	❑	_____
8.	Calculate drug dosage and check calculations with another nurse	❑	❑	_____
9.	Check compatibility chart or consult pharmacy if mixing two medications	❑	❑	_____
10.	Remove metal cap from top of vial; wipe rubber diaphragm briskly with alcohol sponge	❑	❑	_____
11.	Pull plunger of syringe back to aspirate air into syringe equal to amount of drug to be withdrawn	❑	❑	_____
12.	Insert needle into inverted vial; inject air and withdraw volume of solution to be given; keep needle under solution to prevent aspiration of air into syringe	❑	❑	_____
13.	Push plunger gently to disperse solution to tip of needle; remove air bubbles by gently tapping syringe	❑	❑	_____

PERFORMANCE CHECKLIST 22-13B

Preparing Parenteral Medications (con't): Withdrawing Medication from an Ampule

		S	U	Comments
1.	Follow the six rights	❏	❏	_____
2.	Perform the three label checks	❏	❏	_____
3.	Follow standard precautions	❏	❏	_____
4.	Check for allergies	❏	❏	_____
5.	Wash hands before handling equipment; prepare medication in clean area; reduce distractions	❏	❏	_____
6.	Keep sterile parts of syringe and needle sterile; use aseptic technique throughout preparation	❏	❏	_____
7.	Compare drug and dosage ordered with drug and dosage on hand; check expiration date, dosage per milliliter, total volume of solution in ampule; look for contaminants or defects in ampule	❏	❏	_____
8.	Calculate drug dosage and check calculations with another nurse	❏	❏	_____
9.	Check compatibility chart or consult pharmacy if mixing two medications	❏	❏	_____
10.	Tap the top of ampule to move solution from top of ampule to bottom of ampule	❏	❏	_____
11.	Cover neck of ampule with an alcohol sponge, break off top of ampule; deposit top of glass ampule in sharps container	❏	❏	_____
12.	Use a filter needle to aspirate medication from ampule. Filter or aspiration needles catch particles of glass that may be in the solution from the broken ampule	❏	❏	_____
13.	Insert filter needle into open neck of ampule, invert ampule to withdraw correct dose	❏	❏	_____

	S	U	Comments
14. Replace filter needle with needle appropriate for purpose of solution and viscosity of solution	❏	❏	_____
15. Push plunger gently until the medication is at tip of needle	❏	❏	_____

PERFORMANCE CHECKLIST 22-13C

PREPARING PARENTERAL MEDICATIONS (CON'T): RECONSTITUTING A POWDERED DOSAGE FORM

		S	U	Comments
1.	Follow the six rights	❏	❏	_____
2.	Perform the three label checks	❏	❏	_____
3.	Follow standard precautions	❏	❏	_____
4.	Check for allergies	❏	❏	_____
5.	Wash hands before handling equipment; prepare medication in clean area; reduce distractions	❏	❏	_____
6.	Keep sterile parts of syringe and needle sterile; use aseptic technique throughout preparation	❏	❏	_____
7.	Compare drug and dosage ordered with drug and dosage on hand; check expiration date, dosage per milliliter, total volume of solution in vial; look for contaminants or defects in vial	❏	❏	_____
8.	Calculate drug dosage and check calculations with another nurse	❏	❏	_____
9.	Check compatibility chart or consult pharmacy if mixing two medications	❏	❏	_____
10.	Follow instructions on manufacturer's box and drug insert; the instructions will specify the type and amount of diluent to use (for example, add 10 ml bacteriostatic normal saline to prepare a ratio of 500 mg/ml)	❏	❏	_____
11.	Remove the protective cap from diluent; withdraw diluent using sterile technique	❏	❏	_____
12.	Withdraw needle from diluent vial	❏	❏	_____
13.	Inject diluent into vial of powdered drug; gently shake and tap vial to dissolve powder into solution	❏	❏	_____

	S	U	Comments

14. If solution is multidose vial, label solution with:

    a.   Date and time mixed   ❑ ❑ _____

    b.   Name of person who mixed drug and diluent   ❑ ❑ _____

    c.   Dosage per milliliter obtained (concentration)   ❑ ❑ _____

    d.   Amount and type of diluent used   ❑ ❑ _____

15. Withdraw correct dose; select appropriate needle gauge and length for patient   ❑ ❑ _____

PERFORMANCE CHECKLIST 22-13D

PREPARING PARENTERAL MEDICATIONS (CON'T): PLACING TWO MEDICATIONS INTO ONE SYRINGE (INSULIN EXAMPLE USED)

		S	U	Comments
1.	Follow the six rights	❑	❑	_____
2.	Perform the three label checks	❑	❑	_____
3.	Follow standard precautions	❑	❑	_____
4.	Check for allergies	❑	❑	_____
5.	Wash hands before handling equipment; prepare medication in clean area; reduce distractions	❑	❑	_____
6.	Keep sterile parts of syringe and needle sterile; use aseptic technique throughout preparation	❑	❑	_____
7.	Compare drug and dosage ordered with drug and dosage on hand; check expiration date, dosage per milliliter, total volume of solution in vial; look for contaminants	❑	❑	_____
8.	Calculate drug dosage and check calculations with another nurse	❑	❑	_____
9.	Check compatibility of two drugs with a compatibility chart or call pharmacy	❑	❑	_____
10.	Check and compare label of each drug ordered with label of each drug on hand	❑	❑	_____
11.	Compare each label with medication order	❑	❑	_____
12.	Roll long- and intermediate-acting insulin between the palms; do not shake any insulin [note: do not mix long-acting glargine insulin (Lantus) with regular insulin; Lantus insulin is clear and does not need to be rolled to mix; precipitation may occur]	❑	❑	_____
13.	Briskly wipe tops of both vials with separate alcohol swab	❑	❑	_____

	S	U	Comments
14. Pull back plunger of syringe to amount equal to volume of longer-acting insulin to be given	❏	❏	_____
15. Insert needle and inject air into vial of longer-acting insulin	❏	❏	_____
16. Withdraw needle from vial; do not remove insulin	❏	❏	_____
17. Pull back plunger of syringe to amount equal to volume of shorter-acting (regular) insulin to be given	❏	❏	_____
18. Insert needle through rubber stopper of second vial; inject air into vial	❏	❏	_____
19. Invert vial; withdraw volume of shorter-acting (regular) insulin	❏	❏	_____
20. Check and verify dosage in syringe with another nurse against medication order	❏	❏	_____
21. Wipe rubber stopper of longer-acting insulin; insert needle of the syringe containing shorter-acting insulin and withdraw ordered dose of longer-acting insulin. Verify dosage with another nurse	❏	❏	_____
22. Remove needle/syringe from vial	❏	❏	_____
23. Check labels of both vials against medication order	❏	❏	_____
24. Pull plunger back far enough to allow space in barrel of syringe for insulin to be gently mixed; mix by tilting syringe back and forth; remove air	❏	❏	_____
25. Follow procedure for room, bed, and patient identification	❏	❏	_____
26. Give mixed insulin immediately	❏	❏	_____
27. Don gloves	❏	❏	_____
28. Inject subcutaneously	❏	❏	_____
29. Record administration in Medex or computer with site, initials, date, and time	❏	❏	_____
30. Return to assess patient's response to medication	❏	❏	_____
31. Document assessment in nurse's notes	❏	❏	_____

Student Name _____ Date _____ Instructor's Name _____

PERFORMANCE CHECKLIST 22-14

GIVING AN INTRAMUSCULAR INJECTION

		S	U	Comments
1.	Follow the six rights	❏	❏	_____
2.	Perform the three label checks	❏	❏	_____
3.	Follow standard precautions	❏	❏	_____
4.	Wash hands	❏	❏	_____
5.	Check for allergies	❏	❏	_____
6.	Prepare medication according to standard procedure for injectables	❏	❏	_____
7.	Identify room, bed, and patient	❏	❏	_____
8.	Recheck for allergies	❏	❏	_____
9.	Don gloves	❏	❏	_____
10.	Explain the procedure	❏	❏	_____
11.	Recheck for allergies	❏	❏	_____
12.	Select and expose site (according to IM site selection procedure); provide privacy	❏	❏	_____
13.	Clean skin with alcohol swab (from center outward), spread skin tight with thumb and index finger, and let dry	❏	❏	_____
14.	Ask patient to take a deep breath and exhale slowly to relax muscle as needle is inserted (lessens pain from injection)	❏	❏	_____
15.	Insert needle at a 90-degree angle quickly in a dartlike motion; quickness reduces discomfort	❏	❏	_____
16.	Maintain needle in muscle; gently aspirate (pull back plunger) to be certain needle is in muscle and not in a vein or an artery	❏	❏	_____

	S	U	Comments
17. If blood is seen, needle is in a vein or artery; withdraw needle; discard solution; prepare new medication; select another site	❏	❏	_____
18. Slowly inject medication into muscle to lessen discomfort	❏	❏	_____
19. Withdraw needle quickly without bending or twisting it	❏	❏	_____
20. Use pressure and gauze (2 × 2) or Band-Aid to stop any bleeding	❏	❏	_____
21. Do not recap needle (if safety glide needle used, advance protective glide); dispose directly into sharps container	❏	❏	_____
22. Remove gloves and wash hands	❏	❏	_____
23. Chart site used and amount and type of medication (for example, Demerol 50 mg given IM left ventrogluteal); remember, a quick, dartlike insertion followed by slow injection of the medication is much less painful to the patient	❏	❏	_____
24. Record administration in Medex or computer with site, initials, date, and time	❏	❏	_____
25. Return to assess patient's response to medication	❏	❏	_____
26. Document assessment in nurse's notes	❏	❏	_____

PERFORMANCE CHECKLIST 22-15

GIVING A Z-TRACK INJECTION

		S	U	Comments
1.	Follow the six rights	❏	❏	_____
2.	Perform the three label checks	❏	❏	_____
3.	Follow standard precautions	❏	❏	_____
4.	Wash hands	❏	❏	_____
5.	Check for allergies	❏	❏	_____
6.	Prepare medication according to standard procedure for injectables	❏	❏	_____
7.	Identify room, bed, and patient	❏	❏	_____
8.	Recheck for allergies	❏	❏	_____
9.	Don gloves	❏	❏	_____
10.	Use one needle to withdraw dose from container; use another needle (1½ to 2 inches) to inject medication so that no solution remains on the outside needle shaft	❏	❏	_____
11.	Draw up to 0.2 ml of air to create an air lock	❏	❏	_____
12.	Expose and locate dorsogluteal or ventrogluteal site according to IM site selection procedure; provide privacy	❏	❏	_____
13.	Clean site with an alcohol swab	❏	❏	_____
14.	Ask the patient to take a deep breath and to slowly exhale (to relax the muscle); pull skin tightly in a lateral direction (move skin at least 1 to 1½ inch laterally) to one side; hold the skin taut with the nondominant hand	❏	❏	_____
15.	Insert needle at a 90-degree angle; aspirate; if no blood is seen, inject medication and air slowly; wait 10 seconds to allow the medication to disperse slowly	❏	❏	_____

	S	U	Comments
16. Withdraw needle quickly; allow skin to return to its normal position, which leaves a zigzag path that seals the needle track wherever tissue planes slide across each other. The drug cannot escape from the muscle tissue	❏	❏	_____
17. Use a 2 × 2 inch gauze pad or Band-Aid as needed	❏	❏	_____
18. Do not massage site	❏	❏	_____
19. Do not recap needle (if safety glide needle used, advance protective glide); dispose directly into sharps container	❏	❏	_____
20. Remove gloves and wash hands	❏	❏	_____
21. Chart site used, Z-track method used, and amount and type of medication given	❏	❏	_____

Student Name _____ Date _____ Instructor's Name _____

PERFORMANCE CHECKLIST 22-16

GIVING AN INTRADERMAL INJECTION

		S	U	Comments
1.	Follow the six rights	❏	❏	_____
2.	Perform the three label checks	❏	❏	_____
3.	Follow standard precautions	❏	❏	_____
4.	Wash hands	❏	❏	_____
5.	Check for allergies	❏	❏	_____
6.	Prepare medication according to standard procedure for injectables	❏	❏	_____
7.	Recheck for allergies	❏	❏	_____
8.	Don gloves	❏	❏	_____
9.	Identify patient and explain procedure	❏	❏	_____
10.	Recheck for allergies	❏	❏	_____
11.	Select and expose inner aspect of lower arm	❏	❏	_____
12.	Clean site gently with alcohol swab from center outward; let dry	❏	❏	_____
13.	Two injections are made if test is for sensitivity. One injection is a control using sterile water or bacteriostatic normal saline; the other is the substance that is to be tested	❏	❏	_____
14.	Insert a 25-gauge needle at approximately a 15-degree angle with bevel up directly under skin to make a small bleb (wheal) with test solution; do not inject into subcutaneous tissue. Inject control of normal saline into another site for comparison with test substance at designated time interval	❏	❏	_____
15.	Do not massage site	❏	❏	_____

		S	**U**	**Comments**
16.	Draw a circle around skin test with a marker; label area with date, time, and name of test. Another method is to make a diagram in patient's chart to indicate location of site	❏	❏	_____
17.	Do not recap needle (if safety glide needle used, advance protective glide); dispose directly into sharps container	❏	❏	_____
18.	Remove gloves and wash hands	❏	❏	_____
19.	Chart site; intradermal; record initials, date, and time	❏	❏	_____
20.	If an indurated (hardened), erythematous area is observed, measure and record results in millimeters with metric ruler	❏	❏	_____
21.	At designated time, compare control with agent; document results in chart	❏	❏	_____

Student Name _____ Date _____ Instructor's Name _____

GIVING A SUBCUTANEOUS INJECTION

		S	U	Comments
1.	Follow the six rights	❑	❑	_____
2.	Perform the three label checks	❑	❑	_____
3.	Follow standard precautions	❑	❑	_____
4.	Wash hands	❑	❑	_____
5.	Check for allergies	❑	❑	_____
6.	Prepare medication according to standard procedure for injectables	❑	❑	_____
7.	Don gloves	❑	❑	_____
8.	Identify patient and explain procedure	❑	❑	_____
9.	Recheck for allergies	❑	❑	_____
10.	Select and expose site (check which site was used previously and rotate site); the abdomen is the usual preferred site when administering heparin or Lovenox	❑	❑	_____
11.	Clean site with alcohol swab from center outward using circular motion; let dry	❑	❑	_____
12.	Method A: Spread skin of selected site taut and hold firmly; insert needle at 45-degree angle and aspirate; inject medication; do not aspirate if heparin or Lovenox is being administered	❑	❑	_____
13.	Method B: Grasp and press together skin of selected site so that it forms roll between fingers; insert needle at a 90-degree angle and aspirate do not aspirate if heparin or Lovenox is being given; inject medication	❑	❑	_____
14.	Withdraw needle quickly and apply an antiseptic swab or a 2 × 2 inch gauze sponge; do not massage the site if heparin or Lovenox is administered because this will increase local bleeding and ecchymosis will occur	❑	❑	_____

	S	U	Comments
15. Do not recap needle (if safety glide needle used, advance protective glide); dispose directly into sharps container	❏	❏	_____
16. Remove gloves and wash hands	❏	❏	_____
17. Chart site used and amount and type of medication; subcutaneous; record initials, date, and time	❏	❏	_____

Student Name _____ Date _____ Instructor's Name _____

PERFORMANCE CHECKLIST 23-1

APPLYING A TOURNIQUET

		S	U	Comments
1.	Use a strong, wide, flat piece of material if possible (for example, towel, necktie, wide belt)	❏	❏	_____
2.	Place pressure on the nearest pressure point to control bleeding while applying the tourniquet	❏	❏	_____
3.	Apply a pad (piece of cloth, handkerchief, dressing) over the artery to be compressed to prevent impairment of skin integrity	❏	❏	_____
4.	Place the tourniquet between the wound and the heart: allow some uninjured skin between the wound and the tourniquet; wrap the material around the limb twice, and tie a half-knot on the upper surface of the limb	❏	❏	_____
5.	Place a stick or rod (approximately 6 inches long) over the knot, and secure it in place	❏	❏	_____
6.	Twist the stick enough times to stop the bleeding	❏	❏	_____
7.	Secure the stick firmly with the free ends of the tourniquet; do not cover the tourniquet	❏	❏	_____
8.	Write "T" or "TK" (meaning tourniquet) on the victim's forehead and the time it was applied; attach a note to the victim's clothing describing the time and location of the tourniquet	❏	❏	_____
9.	Treat for shock, and transport to the nearest medical facility	❏	❏	_____
10.	Never loosen a tourniquet once it has been applied; always seek medical attention once tourniquet has been applied	❏	❏	_____

Student Name _____ Date _____ Instructor's Name _____

APPLYING AN ARM SPLINT USING A TRIANGULAR SLING AND SWATHE BANDAGE

		S	U	Comments
1.	Place one end of the base of the open triangle over the uninjured shoulder	❏	❏	_____
2.	Place the apex of the triangle behind the elbow of the injured arm	❏	❏	_____
3.	Bend the arm at the elbow with the hand elevated slightly (4–5 inches)	❏	❏	_____
4.	Bring the forearm across the chest and over the bandage	❏	❏	_____
5.	Take the lower end of the triangle, and bring it over the shoulder of the injured side; tie the bandage on the neck at the uninjured side so that the knot is on the side of the neck	❏	❏	_____
6.	Twist the remaining end of the bandage, and tuck it in at the elbow	❏	❏	_____
7.	Remember to keep fingertips exposed to assess circulation	❏	❏	_____

PERFORMANCE CHECKLIST 23-3

MOVING THE VICTIM WITH A SUSPECTED SPINAL CORD INJURY

		S	U	Comments
1.	Carefully roll the victim, supporting the entire length of the body, just enough to slip a solid board underneath the victim for support; this board must extend beyond the victim's head and feet	❑	❑	_____
2.	While another person steadies the victim's head, place a towel or padding in the space underneath the victim's neck (never put the head on a pillow)	❑	❑	_____
3.	Place additional padding (rolled up blankets, towels, sandbags, etc.) around the head and neck to hold the head in place, keeping the neck in line with the body; a cervical collar may be used	❑	❑	_____
4.	Secure the victim to the backboard with bandages, or improvise these so that the entire body is immobilized; tape the head in place	❑	❑	_____
5.	In the event of an emergency situation in which the victim is wearing a helmet, the nurse should immobilize the victim with the helmet left in place	❑	❑	_____

NOTES

NOTES

NOTES

NOTES

NOTES

NOTES

NOTES

NOTES